GW01238519

This book is a self-help gu— problems. It tells what th— eliminate their problems — is not something that must be passively accepted. Just — it is possible to learn to remain awake under special circumstances, it is possible to learn to sleep well again. Dr. Langen, Director of the Clinic and Polyclinic for Psychotherapy at the University Clinic of Mainz, bases his self-help program on these new medical findings.

Step 1: The reader becomes familiar with how the sleep-wakefulness mechanism functions, learns the workings of man's biological clock, and the significance of dreams to sleep.

Step 2: Professor Langen explains how people with sleeping problems can liberate themselves from sleep medications in order to regain the ability to sleep.

Step 3: Various kinds of sleep disturbances, their causes, and treatments are clearly described in detail. By making a record of sleep habits and analyzing it, the patient finds out exactly which type of sleeper he is and can then initiate a planned program of treatment.

Professor Dietrich Langen, M.D.
Born in 1913 in Apia, Samoa. Studied medicine in Munich and Breslau.
Taught from 1958 to 1964 at University of Tuebingen, where he was head physician at the Nerve Clinic. Since 1965, Professor at the University of Mainz. Professor of Psychotherapy and Medical Psychology. Director of Clinic and Polyclinie for Psychotherapy at the University of Mainz. Honorary membership in fourteen international medical societies.

Published by
Sterling Publishers Private Limited

Speaking of:
Sleeping Problems

Dietrich Langen, M.D.

Speaking of:
Sleeping Problems

Learning to Sleep Well Again

Including Directions for Making an Analysis of
Your Sleep and Keeping a Sleep Diary

**In Collaboration with Renate Zauner
Translation: Martha Humphreys**

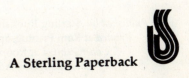

A Sterling Paperback

STERLING PAPERBACKS
An imprint of
Sterling Publishers (P) Ltd.
L-10, Green Park Extension, New Delhi-110016

Speaking of: Sleeping Problems
©1994, Sterling Publishers Pvt. Ltd.
First Indian Edition 1983
Reprint 1987, 1994, 1996

All rights are reserved. No part of this publication may be reproduced, stored in a retrieval system or transmitted, in any form or by any means, mechanical, photocopying, recording or otherwise, without prior written permission of the publisher.

Published by Sterling Publishers Pvt. Ltd., New Delhi-110016.
Printed at Ram Printograph (India), New Delhi-110051.
Cover Printed at Roopak Printer, Delhi-110032.
Cover design by Adage Communications

Contents

1. Sleeping Problems Can Be Avoided

Ability to Sleep Can Be Learned

Many people wonder why sleep is even talked about, because for them sleeping is not a problem and there is no such thing as a sleep disturbance. They sleep well and take sleep for granted. They sleep an hour less or an hour more, just as they at times have more appetite than at others and are sometimes in a good mood, sometimes in a bad mood. They don't check on their sleep, they don't count hours, and they don't compare their sleeping habits with anyone else's. They consider sleep as much a matter of course as digestion. But for many other people, of whom there is an astonishingly large and constantly increasing number in our civilized world, sleep is a problem. These people are always conscious of difficulty in sleeping. They wake up with an almost masochistic satisfaction in saying to themselves, "I knew I couldn't sleep." And they go to bed with the same certainty of, "Again I won't be able to sleep."

Everyone who has trouble sleeping has a strong need for dialogue, for exchanging opinions or sharing experiences with others having similar problems. He does not necessarily look for direct answers to his questions. What he wants is to gain some clarity about himself and his problems, just as many sick persons, after talking to a

11

doctor, then reflect on their problem. This can often be more helpful than medication.

People who have difficulty sleeping are also preoccupied with the problem during the day. Consciously or unconsciously, they consider new regimens, precautions, and medications for the night. They prepare themselves for a sleepless night. They know already in the morning that they will be unable to sleep that night. They get a kind of fixation of considering sleep a problem, and for this reason they eagerly and gratefully adopt all the precautionary measures garnered from others in the same fix. This even includes the exchange of sleeping pills. Later on, they will have to ask their own doctors for a prescription of their own—that is, if the pills have helped. Unfortunately they often do help in the beginning, even though only for a short period of time. As long as the sufferer still has hopes that the medication will be effective, his anxiety about a lack of sleep and his psychic tension abate somewhat, but only for a while. But he makes the mistake of confusing the effects of the medication with his own positive attitude toward sleep. For a short period of time, he has regained his *trust* in *his ability to sleep,* unfortunately through the aid of a false remedy that will soon lose its effectiveness. And after a short phase of disconcertion expressed in a changed ability to sleep, the sufferer is back where he was at the beginning.

Trust in one's own ability to sleep cannot be obtained through medication. It can only be learned through an understanding of the context in which sleep takes place. Sleeplessness is not a permanent condition. The ability to sleep can be regained through a *continuous learning process*. This means that the ability to sleep can be learned, exactly as remaining awake can be learned.

Any person who works as a night nurse, train engineer, doctor, soldier, as an air traffic controller, or as a participant in an expedition learns how to stay awake. This learning process can, however, be reversed and can be applied to the ability to sleep. There is extensive biological proof that it can be done. The most precise formulation about sleep is the statement that among humans sleep is an instinct-related, periodically changing event that, like most other instincts and drives, can to some extent be changed through a learning process.

Sleep As a Drive

Our definition of the influence that learning has on drives is more easily understandable in other areas of human behavior in which drive and instinct are factors. Applied to the drive to eat, it means, for example, that we do not have to eat the very moment we are hungry. We can suppress the drive to eat because we have learned to suppress it. We do not have to give in to an aggressive impulse; we can direct it, suppress it, or divert (transform) it to other impulses. The same applies to the sex drive or to the instinct for danger and protection. Again applied to the drive toward sleep, this means that among humans sleep is instinctual behavior that can be guided by a learning process.

Drives can be redirected by learning processes

Zoologists, biologists, and anthropologists have repeatedly asked why instincts and drives among humans do not have the imperative, absolute quality that they have among animals. The drives toward mating, aggression, hunting, and the chase, for example, all have such imperative status.

Physiologically man is born prematurely

Portmann has attempted the most convincing explanation of this phenomenon. His formulation refers to man's "physiologically premature birth" as the reason that man, in terms of instinct, is the weakest living creature on earth. If the term of pregnancy for the human embryo were comparably as long as among other mammals, pregnancy would have to last two years. If humans were carried to such a term, all sense organs would be fully

13

developed, and the newborn would be able to sit, stand, and walk, would already have bladder control, and would even be somewhat able to speak. He would, as the saying goes, be ready to flee the nest (Portmann).

Since this is not the case, however, maturation among humans must take place outside the uterus. As a result, the human being is exposed during an extremely impressionable time to particularly strong environmental stimuli that have a profound and formative influence on him. Man's instincts and drives are also subject during development to powerful external environmental influence.

In this manner, the human being loses the condition of being imperatively bound to instinct and becomes "open to the world" (Portmann). He is exposed to environmental influences. But this also means that he can learn. The development of the cerebrum, the center of our rational capacities, has not similarly taken place among animals. The possibility of environmental influence is greatly increased by the development of the cerebrum and, as a consequence, what has been learned can also be intellectually understood and retained.

Wrong Sleep Expectation

Exaggerated claims on health

Our expectations or demands concerning health and the smooth and undisturbed functioning of our organism are presumptiously high. We are hardly prepared to make concessions in any area. For example, a headache seems to us to be an imposition, and we reach for pills whenever we have the slightest physical ailment. We can as a matter of course fill our stomachs at any moment with any kind of nourishment. We won't tolerate being thirsty. We can protect ourselves against heat and cold and against any threatening dangers. The level of development of technology in our civilization enables us

14

to afford the incredible luxury of permitting our instincts, which were developed for a life struggle, to atrophy. We have light whenever we need it and a solid roof over our heads, and we seemingly lay claim to solid, deep sleep. We cannot only permit ourselves sleep as a result of our living conditions, we evidently can even buy it at the drugstore.

In fact, no animal sleeps as deeply and firmly as the human. No animal could afford to indulge in such sleep. The neurophysiologist, Jung, even came to ask whether such deep sleep stages as occur among humans, from which people can be awakened only with difficulty, might not be a special by-product of our civilization, since such deep sleep would be extraordinarily risky for an animal living in nature or for a correspondingly unprotected human, as can be confirmed by any war veteran who had to learn to adjust his instinctual sleep behavior to the dangers of the night and of the environment.

Consciously having increasingly estranged ourselves from the biology of our organism and from its basic physiological functions by making night into day, by exercising too little, eating too much, and being overstimulated by the environment, we appeal with high indignation to medicine and the drugstore whenever we are confronted with the consequences of our wrong behavior.

Accepting Being a Short Sleeper

Extremely subjective attitudes and values are usually used in judging one's own sleep. If one spends New Year's Eve among friends, one may go home at three in the morning in an animated and good mood, have a relaxed sleep, and be slightly fatigued the next day without attaching too much importance to the matter. If, however, one lies in bed until 3:00 a.m. without falling

15

asleep, checking the time as it gets later, tossing back a
forth with increasing disquiet, and getting more and mo
nervous, one is exhausted and desperate rather than
animated and in a good mood as on New Year's Eve.
And even if one falls asleep shortly after 3:00 a.m., the
consciousness of having slept little makes one feel wipe
out, tired, dull, and depressed. But in both instances th
amount of sleep is the same; in fact, the hour of falling
asleep is exactly the same. The only difference is in the
evaluation, the initial psychic state, the expectation
concerning sleep, and the subjective judgment about th
lack of sleep. This negative evaluation of one's own sle
increases still more, as a point of comparison, if one's
marital partner is in a deep, quiet sleep. The feeling of
having been short-changed is significantly increased—i
can even climax in aggression—and leads to further
psychological and physical damage.

Subjective evaluation of the amount of sleep

In order to make a judgment about the relation
between the amount of sleep and quality of sleep and t
assess its restorative effect, sleep must be understood
the context of its changing phases, its periodicity, and
involvement with man's biological clock.

Although we spend approximately one-third of our
lives in a sleeping state, little is known about sleep,
because systematic research on the topic has been
conducted only for about forty years, which is the leng
of time instruments have been available for the
evaluation of important findings.

Man spends one-third of his life sleeping

2. What Is Sleep?

A Normal Sleep Pattern

The main difficulty in conducting research on human sleep consists in the sleeper's own inability to provide information about the results of his sleep, so the researcher must use external observation and measurement to the extent possible without disturbing the subject's sleep. If the researcher wakes up the subject, the subject is no longer a sleeper. In fact, the researcher is then at odds with the subject's sleep-wakefulness pattern. The researcher is at the mercy of his own observations concerning sleep. Only since the establishment of well-equipped sleep laboratories and the refinement of the EEG for making brain wave measurements comparable to measurements made by the EKG on the muscular contractions of the heart has it been possible to obtain information about the activities of the brain even during sleep and to develop new insights into the problem.

Rapid eye movement (REM)

Measurements and comparison of brain waves among waking and sleeping persons disclose various patterns, making it possible to distinguish several levels or phases

17

of the depth of sleep that are repeated approximately every two hours during nocturnal sleep. Parallel to these EEG changes, periodically recurring rapid eye movements (abbreviated to REM) can be observed. There are also periodically recurring changes in various vegetative reactions that have an effect on breathing, heartbeat, blood pressure, body temperature, and body movements. The most important results of all these investigations can be approximately summarized as follows:

The depth of sleep changes periodically. During waves of deep sleep in which the body is for the most part calm, there is a buildup of still more important phases of

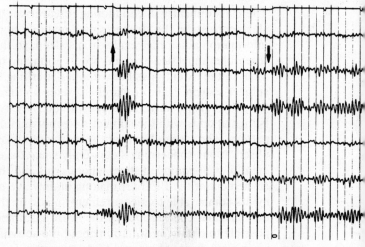

EKG made when subject was slightly tired shows typical alpha rhythm. Compare illustration on page 19.

relative disquiet and lively bodily reactions that are repeated approximately every two hours. The first portion of the slowly increasing depth of sleep with its associated EEG findings is called the "synchronic sleep phase," or "orthodox sleep." It is followed by a significantly contrasting "asynchronic sleep phase," or

18

"paradox sleep," which is called REM sleep because of the strikingly rapid eye movements that occur during it. This asynchronic sleep phase is of critical importance for our health. It is essential to many psychic and physical (psychophysical) processes. We evidently dream during this phase. Just how necessary dream phases are for the well-being of our organism has been shown by experiments in which subjects were deprived of their REM periods. This can be accomplished quite easily by waking up the subject at the start of the rapid eye movements. After being repeatedly deprived of the REM phase, the subject became irritated, discontent, aggressive or even depressed and, if permitted, started to dream with increasing frequency. He seemed to fight for his REM

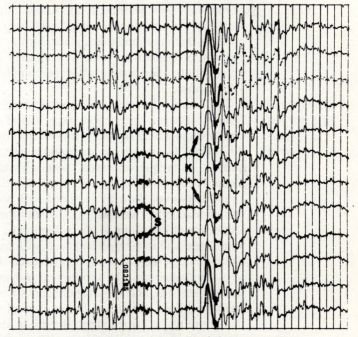

EKG made during a deep sleep stage is clearly different by the absence of the typical alpha rhythm and the presence of sleep spindles (S) and K complexes.

19

phases, and seemed to want to make up for them and to supplement them. Hence it is known that the body does not accept a shortage of REM phases without protest. It makes up for a deficit of REM periods by having more REM periods. French literature therefore mentions a particular form of sleep disturbance characterized by shortened REM phases, using the term "unsuccessful" or "missed" REM periods. Both terms stress the special importance of REM periods.

The pattern of brain wave trackings shows that the periodicity of deep sleep phases steadily becomes smoother during the course of the night. In other words, the separate deep sleep phases become increasingly calm The REM phases do just the opposite. During the course of the night their periodicity increases. They occur more frequently and for longer periods. All subjects tested confirm that dreaming takes place during the REM periods. Subjects were able to recall their dreams immediately upon arousal after the completion of an REM phase.

The course of a normal sleep pattern
The course of normal sleep can be described as follows: it begins with a first stage, a kind of sleepiness, a condition in which contact with the environment is diminished but which can easily be penetrated by arousal stimuli. As fatigue increases, there is a stage of light sleep. Although EEG tracings show that the brain is already involved during this period with real sleep, it can still be reached by external stimuli. But these stimuli no longer result in waking up the subject, i.e., sensory stimuli are still registered and dealt with by the appropriate sense organ but do not reach the conscious-ness for evaluation. The subsequent transition to deep sleep is smooth, and the sleeper cannot easily be awakened from this phase. In fact, not all sleepers reach this phase to the same extent; the phase also varies in duration, but it is a part of normal sleep. This rhythm is repeated approximately five or six times within one night The pattern of the curve becomes increasingly smooth

20

while, as already described, the dream phases occurring at intervals in between become longer, more frequent, and more intensive.

Deviations from the Sleep Norm

Phase shifts resulting from sleep disturbances

Various phases of this normal sleep pattern can be affected by sleep disturbances. For example, the time that elapses before the beginning of the first deep sleep phase can be lengthened, and the first REM phase can be incomplete (unsuccessful REM sleep). And instead of the normal cyclic leveling-off into deep sleep, an interval of complete wakefulness can occur, thereby shortening the total sleep time and having a subjective effect on the feeling of restoration in the morning. In addition, the quantitative relation between synchronic and asynchronic REM sleep seems to be important. And, finally, the entire cyclic succession of the separate phases can be jumbled up, which occurs in severe mental illness.

Errors in estimating amount of time slept

Brain wave tracings documenting experiments conducted in the sleep laboratory have revealed still other findings of importance to persons with sleep problems. One is the evident difficulty in judging one's own sleep. Many test subjects who indicated that they had only thought about something but had not slept had in reality dreamed. They did not perceive the duration of light sleep periods and gave false estimates of the duration of intervals of wakefulness. This shows that disturbances of this periodic event are subjectively overrated and are experienced far more strongly than indicated by objective findings. Hence the impression of not having slept the whole night is often demonstrably false. But since the morning feeling of restoration is largely based on an awareness of the amount of sleep, it is understandable why the feeling of difficulty in sleeping can be so strong despite an objectively sufficient amount of sleep. The

21

reason is that it is almost impossible to judge one's own sleep without special equipment. The idea that one has usually slept more than one thought should therefore provide some comfort, because the body in any case gets the minimal quantity of sleep needed.

The sleep periods—i.e., the two-hour rhythmic course of the various sleep phases—account for why it is so difficult to fall asleep again if the first deep sleep is interrupted. A new high point of fatigue simply does not occur until two hours later, and there is really not much sense in trying to force sleep against this biological rhythm, because the body just will not cooperate. In such an instance, it is better to wait for a new period of fatigue, perhaps to fill the interval by reading, and to give in and wait for the organism's next demand for sleep, which will occur with the next drop in the synchronic sleep curve.

The right time for falling back to sleep

The fact that other bodily functions also change in response to the particular stage of sleep has already been mentioned. These include in particular the heart rate, blood pressure, frequency and depth of breathing, and therefore the supply of oxygen to the blood, dilation of the pupils, perspiration, and excitation of the sex organs. We will later see that this linkage of sleep periods to the autonomic nervous system also often gives us the opportunity of positively influencing sleep in the regulation of these mechanisms (see page 88). These events also support the contemporary definition of sleep as an active accomplishment of the organism resulting in extensive changes in bodily processes.

The Sleep-Wakefulness Mechanism

Attempts at anatomically localizing sleep in the brain gained increasing importance in sleep research, and efforts were made to discover which areas of the brain govern sleeping and waking. Biochemistry similarly undertook the investigation of possible endogenous sleep-releasing substances. The idea of eventually coming upon an endogenous substance that could be isolated and that would dependably be able to induce physiological sleep of a chosen amount holds great fascination. After all, annual consumption of soporifics and tranquillizers in the Western countries alone is measured in tons.

In the process of experimentation, through stimulation of certain areas of the brain, it was in fact possible in experiments on animals to make out certain zones (somnogenous zones) in the mid-brain which when stimulated triggered states resembling sleep. It was similarly possible in other areas of the mid-brain to delineate so-called "waking centers." After the discovery of still other zones of the mid-brain relevant to the sleep-wakefulness mechanism—especially after the discovery of a brain structure extending from the medulla oblongata to the mid-brain, the *formatio reticularis*—interest was focused on the sleep-wakefulness mechanism that regulates the sleep-waking cycle. Present knowledge about this mechanism is as follows:

Nerve structures direct the sleep-waking cycle

The sleep-wakefulness mechanism functions within a whole system of stimulating (activating), subduing, and diffuse nerve structures that cannot be precisely delineated. In part, these nerve structures are symmetrically laid out, and they extend from the upper end of the spine in the medulla oblongata across the mid-brain, and partially extend into the different areas of the cerebrum. This system of nerve structures, in addition to aiding the sleep-wakefulness mechanism, also assists in activating or subduing mental processes and movement (motoricity) and in regulating the autonomic nervous system that influences all these events.

No specific sleep center in the brain

The significance of this knowledge consists in the realization that there is no sleep center in the brain that acts in an isolated manner. Either it functions, in which case we can sleep; or it doesn't function, in which case

23

we need sleeping pills. It is more accurate to state that the brain is a central organ that affects the entire organism. It constantly emits stimulating or subduing impulses that direct the functioning and activity within the organism. Areas affected include active body movements, functions within the autonomic nervous system, regulation of the functioning of the organs, breathing, circulation, sleep-wakefulness mechanism, and mental activity. In this manner, all these processes are influenced and *centrally controlled*. The most important characteristic shared by these brain structures is therefore a *unity* determined by *function*.

Bodily functions are centrally controlled

In terms of anatomy, the occipital parts of these brain structures have greater control over wakefulness, the frontal parts have greater control over sleeping. This cannot be viewed in an isolated manner, however. Similar to the feedback control system of a thermostat, it is the interaction that keeps us in the realm of normalcy.

Man's Biological Clock

If persons are so shut off from the outer world that they have no external time-markers such as light, sound, or other changes that admit inferences to social life (as, for example, in the bunker experiments made by Ashoff), the surprising result among a majority of test subjects is that their biological clocks are oriented toward a 24-hour rhythm over long periods of time.

The biological sense of time

The 24-hour rhythm is caused by the rotation of the earth and the resulting alternation of light and darkness. But, surprisingly enough, the biological periodicity of animals and humans is not precisely fitted to this cycle. Actually the periodicity mostly shows a somewhat longer rhythmic pattern lasting about 25 hours, or occasionally even a shorter rhythmic period lasting about 23.5 hours. Only rarely is it shorter than 23.5 hours. In this context,

24

Halberg spoke of circadian periodicity, which is derived from "circa," meaning "approximately," and "dian," meaning "corresponding to the day." In other words, circadian means related to the 24-hour cycle. Biological periodicity, which is oriented toward a 24-hour cycle, is a fixed rhythmic pattern. The cycle is in fact frequently longer than 24 hours, only rarely shorter, but it determines our biological feeling for time.

There are species of animals whose inner clocks are oriented toward rhythms other than the alternation between darkness and light. For example, the time-marker among many crabs and mussels is the ocean s tidal change, a 12 ¾-hour cycle, as the tide is a more important factor than light in the life of these species.

Biologi-cally-determined long and short sleep-ers

Hence it may be stated that biological clocks vary to some extent according to species. Birds, for example, have a differently oriented biological clock than fish, and fish in turn have a differently oriented biological clock than man. Within the species, however, there are early risers and late sleepers. Experiments with chaffinches (Aschoff) confirm this observation. Comparable to early risers among humans, birds used in the experiment started flying 1.5 hours before the light stimulus was turned on to wake them up. Other birds in the experiment only began to fly .5 hours after the light signal. In other words, they had a longer circadian cycle than the early risers, and although there is a biological clock peculiar to the species chaffinch, even among them there are individual short sleepers and long sleepers.

The sleep-wakefulness mechanism is not the only function controlled by the biological clock. All other vegetatively controlled bodily functions and many aspects of psychic behavior are also subject to this rhythm. The functioning of our own circadian periodicity can be observed even by the medical layman whenever there are any sudden, short-term changes in the accustomed time system such as occurs in flying east or west. Our biological clock requires several 24-hour cycles to regain its normal course and adjust to a new time system. Readjusting (resynchronization) usually takes longer on flights to the west than to the east. In addition, individual vegetatively controlled organic systems require varying periods of time for resynchronization. If the biological clock has not yet completely adjusted to the new time, both mental and physical efficiency is significantly impaired. For this reason, after longer east-west flights people should immediately allow for a rest of at least several hours to give their biological clocks some opportunity to adjust to the local time in the new setting.

The discrepancy between our biological clock, which has a rhythm of approximately 25 hours, and the 24-hour rhythm of our day and night cycle constantly compels us to reconcile the difference. Our sleep rhythm must also actively participate in this ongoing process of adjustment. The necessity of the sleeper to learn to adjust provides biological proof that life means, among other things, learning to overcome discrepancies or ostensible deviations.

The Biochemistry of Sleep

The biochemistry of sleep is still to a large extent in the stage of experimentation and speculation. For this reason, we only wish to touch on this subject now. We still know relatively little about the topic, despite the fact that there is a great deal of interest in research on the subject, because of the extreme difficulty in obtaining and analyzing such rapidly occurring chemical events in such complicated structures as that of the central nervous system.

A series of substances that are important in transmitting impulses are already known, and these substances are involved in any event controlled by the nerves.

26

Acetylcholin, serotonin, and noradrenalin are several of these transmitter substances (neurohormones) involved in transmitting stimuli in the central nervous system. Serotonin seems to be of special importance for deep sleep. In any case, substances that impede the formation of serotonin in the organism result in sleeplessness in experiments, while noradrenalin seems to be more responsible for the REM phases of sleep. But these matters are to a large extent hypotheses that we do not wish to go into further at this point.

3. Subjective and Objective Quality of Sleep

Amount of Sleep and Need for Sleep

Everyone troubled with difficulty in sleeping is accustomed to keeping exact records of the number of hours slept. While it is easy to keep track of time with the aid of a clock, it is far more difficult to measure mental states or feelings of contentment. The reason for keeping such records is because of a subjective expectation concerning sleep, especially the amount of time slept. The quality of sleep is less tangible and is more difficult to measure and assess.

Another psychological factor is at work, however, in this need for an exact record—the unstated comparison with the healthy sleeper and with an established sleep norm. People with sleep problems often have the erroneous idea that normal sleep results from a physiological need to sleep a specific number of hours and is the condition for conveying the subjective feeling of "having slept enough" or of "having had a good night's rest."

Presumed sleep norms

The notion of a specific quantity of sleep is related to the idea of its restorative effect. Thoughts are automatically paired, and much sleep is equated with feeling fresh, feeling rested is equated with a capacity for work. Conversely, a little amount of sleep is equated with

29

tiredness, dullness, and inefficiency.

It has already been mentioned how difficult it is for the poor sleeper to judge the length of time slept. But it is the poor sleeper who makes astonishingly exact notations of the times he "didn't sleep at all," including detailed calculations of the hours and minutes. It would be very tempting once to put such assertions of "not having slept at all" to a test in a sleep laboratory to demonstrate that many of the periods that seem to the poor sleeper to be waking periods are in reality dream phases or stages of light sleep. It could be shown, too, that several short sleep periods do amount to real sleep, even though perhaps only to a small amount of sleep.

Many problem sleepers simply have difficulty in accepting their individual condition of being short sleepers. They cannot resist making constant comparisons with the seemingly normal sleepers in their vicinity and confronting themselves with what they believe to be their own sleep deficit. The eight-hour norm regrettably accepted by so many people as standard is as untenable as prescribing a generally valid amount of food to be consumed by everyone or as establishing a norm for sexual behavior.

The errone-
ous 8-hour
norm

In addition, it seems altogether possible that the characteristics of a person's sleep are partially an inherited tendency.

Inherited
tendencies
toward
sleep

Research with families have revealed certain types of sleepers, short sleepers and long sleepers. If the short sleeper has the possibility of investigating the question, he may find that even as a child he was always considered a mischief-maker who was forever awake, could hardly be brought to take the usual morning or afternoon nap, was awake in the evening, and full of life in the morning. If an infant who was only accustomed to sleeping ten hours were able to suspect himself of being short sleeper, he would be horrified to compare his own sleep record with that of other infants in the vicinity who sleep 15 to 18 hours a day.

30

The most well-known short sleepers of all time, Edison and Napoleon, are repeatedly quoted as having gotten along on two hours of sleep. Edison is reputed to have discovered the light bulb in order that man should not have to waste so much valuable time in his life by sleeping. Napoleon's sleep habits prove that periods of great activity by no means required being offset by periods of much sleep. On the contrary, during periods of great activity and efficiency, it is sometimes possible to get along with very little sleep. Certainly the need for sleep is evidently very different among different individuals, and many an alledged sleep disturbance is the result of not knowing one's own sleep requirements. Therefore fatigue and exhaustion are to a large extent the result of a psychic reaction to what is perceived as a lack of sleep and would be much less frequent complaints if many people simply accepted the fact that they are four- or five-hour sleepers.

Need for sleep varies individually

An additional factor is that when there is a lack of sleep, the sleep periods missed vary in importance to the organism, depending upon when they occurred, since other bodily functions adjust to the wavy, rhythmic course of sleep. If the autonomic nervous system just happens to be in a phase of excitation, it can make a waking phase very disagreeable through such manifestations as heart palpitation, anxiety, and perspiration. Because of the readiness for deep sleep in the hours after midnight, a waking period around this time will result in a minimal feeling of being refreshed and restored and a maximal feeling of fatigue and exhaustion. If the person remains awake, sleepiness diminishes with the approach of morning and the feeling of being refreshed and capable of activity increases even though the organism was unable in the interval to be restored by additional sleep. For this reason, a period of being awake shortly after midnight is subjectively more serious and depressing than a period of being awake toward morning. By the time morning approaches, one's whole mood is better,

Importance of when sleep interruptions occur

31

enabling one to make a more positive evaluation of one'
own state and the approaching new day. Even the
low point at a big dance is biologically predictable to be
around 2:00 a.m. Conversely, most people feel physiolc
ically revived toward morning.

The amount of sleep registered by one person as
normal can therefore be registered by another person
with the feeling of a torturous sleeplessness.

*Quality of
sleep and
feeling of
recuperation*

But the feeling of restoration, apart from the psychic
evaluation just described, is also dependent upon the
quality of sleep, i.e., it is dependent upon the various
sleep phases, their length, and the order in which they
occur. Moreover, the often satisfying feeling of "I have
slept" seems to be particularly related to the periodic
alternation between synchronic and asynchronic sleep
periods. If this alternation is absent, there is no feeling
recuperation. We will discuss this fact again in
connection with the use of sleeping pills (see page 68).

A comparison of laboratory sleep records of long
sleepers and short sleepers, both of which groups
consider themselves normal sleepers, shows that the
decisive factor in the restorative effect of sleep is not t.
amount of sleep but the maintenance of certain sleep
phases. Evidently some sleep phases can be dispensed
with. Consequently both types of sleepers can have
approximately the same number of deep sleep phases,
including REM phases, but can vary in the intervals of
light sleep or the respective length of the separate slee
phases. The transitional phases of light sleep can in fac
be completely missing among short sleepers without
producing the feeling of having had an insufficient
amount of sleep. The short sleeper simply sleeps more
concentratedly, to some extent "faster."

*Relation be-
tween
dream and
deep sleep
phases*

The general maintenance of a certain relation betwe
the totality of the dream phases and the other sleep
periods seems to be important for achieving the greate
perceptible restorative effect. But it cannot be proved
which form of sleep is more desirable, short deep slee

32

long even sleep. It is therefore impossible to assign any exact normal values for the length of time slept. The range of variation is from five to ten hours. But even this statement represents values that can vary in either direction.

Total sleep deprivation

What happens, though, if sleep is totally withheld? Numerous experiments of immense value to problem sleepers have been made in the course of years by volunteer test subjects. This should be constantly kept in mind if you become nervous and desperate in the course of a sleepness night when thinking about greeting the next day with a lack of sleep. Man can tolerate being without sleep for longer periods than is generally imagined. From experiments in complete sleeplessness, the records show periods longer than 200 hours. The longest record is alledgedly held by a 17-year old student from San Diego who managed to spend 264 hours without sleeping. Admittedly he did not work during that period of time, which amounts to 11 days and nights!

As already mentioned, though, complete lack of sleep occurs only in an experimental situation when the subject is effectively impeded even from the slightest attempt at sleep. Under normal conditions, the organism obtains the minimal quantity of sleep needed, even if in very small,

Body se- ures mini- mal quan- y of sleep

subjectively hardly noticeable intervals. The body is able, however, to make up in one night for even a long sleepless period. In other words, the regenerative capacity is extraordinarily great, at least in this area.

Sleep among Infants and the Elderly

An infant is known to sleep considerably more than a mature person. However, even at this early age there are differences in the need for sleep and in the amount of sleep. The number of hours needed can even vary between ten and thirty-two. Many sleep difficulties that later trouble adults can have their origin in infancy.

Pedagogi-
cally
false insis-
tence on
sleep

An infant who is a short sleeper, for example, if coerced to sleep by parents in the erroneous belief that an infant must after all sleep 20 hours, can acquire even at such an early age a complex about being unable to sleep. The child is simply subjected to being trained against its individual biological clock and, in effect, is taught to regard sleep as a problem.

In the beginning, a newborn baby wakes up only when it is hungry, wet, cold, or when it is otherwise disturbed. This condition, called "wakefulness of necessity," (Kleitman) has been contrasted with "wakefulness by choice." As the cerebrum develops, the child learns with increasing regularity to do his sleeping at night, to adjust to the rhythm of the social life of his environment, and to remain awake during the day.

The sleep-wakefulness rhythm is evidently the result of an inborn physiological, periodically changing cycle of activity. Even among adults this cycle is manifested in variations in the degree of feeling awake during the day, mental alertness, and bodily (physical) efficiency.

Young
people's
practice of
shifting day
into night

A familiar practice among young people is the tendency to shift the day-night rhythm toward the direction of late night hours or even toward the early morning hours. Interestingly enough, this can especially be observed among vivid dreamers. The habit conceals dangers, however, which mainly consist in diminished mental productivity and an impaired ability to concentrate. Thinking really requires a rested brain. The assertion of greater mental efficiency during the evening and night hours so often made by students after having shifted day into night (advancing) can at best be supported by the observation there is less distraction and disturbance at night than during the day. For the rest, however, the assertion is a fallacy.

Napping
among the
elderly

Among older persons, the time spent in sleep is significantly shortened, and the character of sleep also changes. The elderly person sleeps less and more superficially, and he does more napping. While the relation between synchronic and asynchronic sleep among infants amounts to 50%, this relation increasingly changes during different phases of life, and among the elderly the REM portion of sleep only amounts to 14%.

Aging, among other things, is also a question of the regulatory capability of the vascular system and is therefore related to the elasticity and condition of the walls of the blood vessels. Leo Buerger, a doctor famous for having conducted research in vascular diseases, made the statement more than 50 years ago that "a person is as old as his blood vessels." It may be assumed that changes in sleep brought about by age are related to these changes in the blood vessels (arteriosclerosis), particularly to the weakening of the elasticity of the vessels in the brain (cerebralsclerosis). It is important to know this—for one reason, because there are far more elderly people than in earlier generations and, for another reason, because of the widespread habit of eagerly and swiftly reaching for sleeping pills.

*Artio-
sclerosis
and sleep*

One of the most essential components of sleep-inducing medications on the market is barbituric acid. In addition to its welcome characteristic of inducing sleep, it has the problematic side effect of lowering the blood pressure and consequently of supplying areas in which circulation is already weak with even less blood and oxygen. In this context, we wish to recall a phenomenon already mentioned in an earlier passage—namely, that during the night the functioning of organs periodically changes. For example, the pulse frequency changes, and so does perspiration, depth and frequency of breathing, and the blood pressure becomes lower. With these changes in mind, it then becomes understandable why a sleeping pill containing barbiturate acid can have an absolutely disastrous effect on an older person. The chain reaction is as follows: as a result of a sclerosis of old age, there is a lack of circulation within the brain, a condition, aggravated both by the diminished strength of the heart as a result of age and by the physiological lowering of the

blood pressure during the night. A single additional
sleeping pill containing barbituric acid then suffices to
decrease the supply oxygen to the brain to such an extent
that the elderly person can become confused and
disoriented, even experience clouding of consciousness
(delirious).

The most sensible recommendation to elderly persons
having difficulty in sleeping, first of all, is to have a
medical consultation to check coronary circulation and
the supply of blood to the brain. Then, instead of
obtaining a prescription for sleeping pills, it may be
indicated that a cardiac stimulant should be taken to
improve circulation and medication prescribed to stimulate the flow of blood through the brain. In many

instances, a cup of coffee drunk before going to bed,
seemingly a "paradox sleep medication," can have a
splendid effect.

An explanation to the elderly about the nature and
amount of sleep as related to age can be of significant
help to them in sleeping by dispelling wrong sleep
expectations and by promoting the acceptance of dozing
off for shorter intervals. Naps, too, taken frequently by
the older person during the course of the day, whether
after eating, while reading the newspaper or looking at
TV, count as sleep. They lessen fatigue at night and
diminish the need for sleep. An increasing lack of
movement and physical exertion among the elderly also
contribute to their need for less sleep than younger
persons have or at least should have. In fact, many sleep
difficulties have their origin in a lack of movement and of
physical fatigue and in the absence of demarcation
between day and night. If someone has already had that
first little bit of sleep lying down in the front of the TV, it
should not be astonishing if he is wide awake after getting
into bed, particularly if we recall the organism's
periodically changing readiness to sleep during the night.
The first opportunity to fall asleep has already been used
during the nap in front of the TV, so there is no

36

alternative but to wait for the next wave of fatigue.

If the person is aware of this, it will certainly be possible to wait with more composure for the moment of falling asleep without reacting abnormally to being awake at night, and the elderly can learn to accept changes in sleep patterns that come with age.

4. Dreaming as Part of Sleep

Dream Phases—Their Biological Necessity

Evidence from prehistoric times to the present confirms that man has always dreamed: In fact, since the time the human brain has slept, man has dreamed. Dreams have always been significant or even uncanny and cause us to do or not to do certain things. One of the oldest and most comprehensive documents on dreams is the *Chester Beathey Papyrus 3* dating from 2000 to 1790 B.C., which describes 2,000 dreams and even rates them as favorable or unfavorable in terms of the dreamer's future. Topics recorded show an astonishing similarity to topics of contemporary dreams and include such significant themes as birth, death, possession, loss, aggressiveness, and occasionally even sexuality. The Assyrians also documented dream fixations, and the Greeks, Romans, and Hebrews took over the animistic concepts of neighboring ethnic groups and adopted the methods of dream interpretation used by the Egyptians and Assyrians (Diamont).

In other words, evidence from the prehistoric era reveals a preoccupation with dreams. The scientific era in the field of sleep research is opened up in the twentieth century. Extensive collections of dreams were made, especially in the United States, and the first significant findings in the field of sleep research included the discovery of the rapid eye movements (REM) that occur during sleep. This led in turn to the earlier mentioned findings (page 18) about the synchronic and asynchronic phases of sleep. A short time later, a connection was made between the asynchronic sleep phase and dreaming.

Diamont describes his observations of these events as follows: ". . . evidently something emotional and exciting was going on simultaneously in the sleeping brain." Kleitman then had the brilliant idea, which he initially just called a hypothesis, that the sleepers were dreaming. He decided to test his assumption by attempting, as has already been described, to arouse test subjects.

These historically significant findings were then published in a short article in the journal, "Science," of September 4, 1953. Twenty-seven arousals during the REM phase provided detailed descriptions of 20 dreams. As a control check on the reliability of the REM phase as an indicator for dreaming, there were 23 arousals when no rapid eye movements were visible. In 19 instances, the sleepers were unable to recall a single dream (Diamont). On the basis of these experiments, Kleitman made the first description of the sleep-dream curve.

Further findings, especially those made by Dement, who was already a scientific colleague of Kleitman while still a medical student, resulted in long-term research, and finally there were 2,500 monitored hours in the first test series available for evaluation. As a result, it was possible to determine the relation between the time spent sleeping and the time spent dreaming. It was shown that the total time spent in sleep by numerous middle-aged test subjects amounted to an average of 7 hours and 2 minutes and that the total time spent dreaming amounted to 82 minutes, or about 20% of the night (see illustration, page 41).

Relation between time spent in sleeping and in dreaming

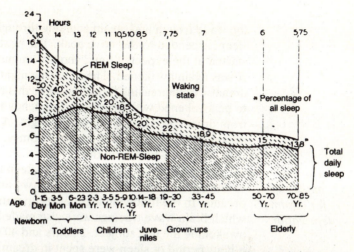

Schematic portrayal of the total number of hours slept in relation to REM sleep, showing the relevance of age to REM sleep. Total amount of sleep and REM sleep diminish with increasing age. Changes occuring in the course of children's maturation are particularly striking.

For the first time, it became abundantly clear that night after night a series of dreams takes place, regardless of whether or not we are able to recall them.

What happens when dreaming is effectively impeded was already covered in the description of the REM phase of sleep and in the explanation of their significance (see page 18). Since Dement's experiments contain such vivid descriptions, they are again included here in some detail. Some volunteer test subjects were permitted first to spend several nights in the sleep laboratory in order to become accustomed to being there. Their sleep behavior was then observed and recorded. Special attention was given to the synchronic and asynchronic sleep phases. The occurrence of dreaming was then impeded for five nights. Test subject A, to be quoted later, was impeded from dreaming for seven nights. Therefore, when A later fell asleep, the EEG showed that a new sleep cycle began immediately, which went through all phases of sleep to

41

the wave trough and, again coursing through all phases of sleep, ascended to the wave peak. The next dream phase started at the expected time, about 90 minutes later, and A was again awakened. The following night, A tried to dream with increasing frequency. For this reason, he had to be awakened with increasing frequency to impede him from dreaming. During the second night, A attempted to dream 10 times, in the third night 17 times, in the fourth night 21 times. Finally in the seventh night it was

The body makes up for dream deprivation

necessary to awaken him 24 times to keep him from dreaming, because A tried to launch two dozen different dreams. In the following night of recuperation, during which brain wave tracings were also made but without awakening the test subject, 2 hours and 40 minutes of an 8-hour period of sleep were spent in dreaming, i.e., one-third of the night, or almost twice the usual amount. The same was repeated during the second night of recuperation. The unavoidable conclusion was that A experienced REM rebound, which means that he made up for dream deprivation by doubling the amount of time spent in dreaming. As a rule in these experiments, after four or five nights of dream deprivation, dreaming increased for about five nights.

The neces-sity of dreaming

These decisive experiments clearly revealed the necessity of dreaming. Every person requires a relatively constant amount of time for dreaming in order for sleep to be restorative. Serious disturbances can otherwise result.

Manifestations occurring during consistent dream deprivation parallel to an astonishing extent the findings of Canadian research in sensory deprivation. These findings show that if sensory impressions are withheld from a person for a certain period of time, the result is confusion in sensory perceptions and ultimately hallucinations.

Although very thorough and extraordinarily comprehensive research has in the meantime been conducted on the relation between REM phases and dream stages,

42

some reasons must be given for not making a too schematic equation between the REM stage and dreaming (Rieger). For one thing, there is no real proof that dreaming does not also take place during the synchronic, deep sleep phase. It is possible that some mental activity is present during this period but that it simply cannot be recalled, just as a large number of "non-dreamers" are unable to recall a single dream immediately after the conclusion of an REM phase. According to all our knowledge of the function of the brain, it must also be assumed that the activity of the cerebral cortex is necessary for the creation of dreams having concrete optic-motor content—i.e., dreams having pictures and action. But we also find REM phases, even particularly abundant REM phases, among newborn infants and animals whose cerebral cortex is not sufficiently developed to differentiate, assimilate, and reproduce optical impressions in a dream. Since a newborn baby, unlike an adult, is not able even in a waking state to stare at objects, the interpretation that would otherwise probably be accurate—that the rapid eye movements result from dream pictures—cannot be supported. Even a person blind from birth who cannot have visual dreams manifests typical REM phases. Even a cat whose cerebral cortex has been removed through an operation and which can surely no longer dream still shows the REM phases with their characteristic lively eye movements, cessation of muscle tension, muscle quivering, and changes in the heart, circulation, and respiration. What we define and measure as the REM periods of sleep are therefore already present (preformed) early in the individual development of the human and in the phylogeny of mammals. The dream, however, only begins to fill this physiological development with content when differentiated functions of consciousness become possible. More simply expressed, dreaming does not bring about the REM phase, but the REM phase seems to some extent to be a condition for dreaming (Rieger).

REM phase
is condition
for dream-
ing

43

There is in all of this some comforting knowledge for problem sleepers. Even short dream periods usually occ during what seems to be a long, sleepless night. The bo simply cannot do without these dream periods and is evidently able to get them, even against considerable obstacles, for they constitute a regenerative process an provide a feeling of recuperation. If one has learned, perhaps by means of autogenic training, to be quiet, doesn't get nervous, and relies on the short, dependabl occurring dream phases, a sleepless night can be passe without, relatively speaking, any ill effect. Even a sleepless night offers rest and REM periods, which are the most important elements of sleep. It is possible mentally to come to terms with a sleepless night, and tl subjective feeling of being rested is measurably increased.

Dream Content

Freudian method of dream interpretation

In response to the question of what determines the con tent of dreams, there are two possibilities of interpretation: the first uses the method developed by Freud of permitting the patient to relate ideas concerning parts c the dream in order to conjecture what the latent, hidde meaning of the dream might be. Anyone familiar with t various interpretations of one and the same dream mad by different analysts has an idea of the suggestive valu of such a procedure. Therefore, the method used in contemporary dream research of investigating the man fest dream content is probably more useful for a scient interpretation of dreams. This latter method is called "immediate interpretation." If the dream series of one night is recorded—usually about five dreams—by arou: ing the sleeper immediately after each dream and lettin him report the dream, the series offers a good opportunity for immediate interpretation. The themes,

'Immediate dream interpretation" method

44

turns out, usually concern utterly serious emotional questions despite the elements of comedy present in dream scenes. In this manner, nocturnal dramas can be reproduced and explained on the basis of their serious background without much subjective interpretation. All that is needed is one or, under certain circumstances, several separate dream series. This kind of investigation is a rewarding field for future research. Direct dream interpretation has the advantage of making it possible to dispense with the dreamer's personal experience, which is of great advantage for an objective judgment, considering how rapidly a patient being treated for mental illness begins to direct dreams toward the doctor. Material from other interpersonal relationships are also involved, so the opinion pollster's technique of "selective listening" used when too many interviews have been gathered is also necessary.

The question still remaining at present is who is responsible for the itinerary of such a dream sequence. Is the topic inner conflict or external conflict? And who or what is involved when there is not present any dynamically operative framework of conflict? So the question could be asked, who is directing the theatrical show of this sequence of dreams that unfolds every night?

Recalling dreams

On the other hand, the question of who recalls his dream can be answered more clearly. In normal sleep, only the last dream that took place before spontaneous awakening is remembered. This is true even if the awakening occurs during the night. Or alternatively the last dream before waking up in the morning is the one remembered. There will be many readers who thought until now that they did not dream at all. From now on, though, they will know that they, too, dream but just don't recall their dreams. So who is who?

It is now necessary to refer again to dream experiments conducted by Diamont. These experiments aided in revealing the difficulty a person has in judging a given,

momentary degree of wakefulness, the transition to
sleep, or the beginning of his own dream. Even those te
subjects who had asserted that they did not dream coul
clearly be observed dreaming. And if they were
awakened at the right moment, they provided detailed
reports of their dreams. Nonetheless, the experiments
revealed two quite subtle differences between the two
groups, the dreamers and the professed non-dreamers.
For one thing, the non-dreamers seemed to have a
mistaken understanding of their dreams. One such
sleeper reported upon being aroused during a period of
REM sleep, that he had been thinking in his sleep. Oth
were unable to decide whether they had thought, slept,
dreamed. In their own words, ". . . I don't know
whether I dream or not. I am not certain whether I hav
slept or not. I had in mind a vision, that I was traveling
down a broad avenue. There was no story, but I was
moving as if I were sitting in a car and the various hou
and building passed by . . . a vision. I can have though
that or dreamed it." And another subject, who initially
showed the same uncertainty in his own judgment, the
came to a different conclusion. ". . . I am not certain
whether I fell asleep . . . I think, though, that I must h
slept. I wouldn't have thought about it if I had been
awake. I cannot imagine it. I believe I must have
dreamed . . ."

One psychological reason for forgetting dreams is
evidently a question of definition. Some non-dreamers
simply do not know what a dream is. Another perhaps
more important reason for forgetting dreams, at least
among alledged non-dreamers, could be that it is more
difficult to arouse them during their dream periods tha
is to arouse the admitted dreamers. The subjects who
difficult to arouse have, compared with other subjects,
few or no dreams at all to report. However, if the
intensity of the arousal signal is increased—for examp
if the bell is rung louder—then immediately after the
louder arousal signal there is a higher percentage of

46

remembered dreams. A sleeper can, therefore, evidently be surprised in such a manner that he has no time to forget his dream (Diamont).

Why dreams are not remembered

Summarizing the question of whether dreams can be recalled, the question must be precisely formulated. At present it can be answered as follows: persons who fall asleep quickly—and they are mostly persons who like to sleep—are as a rule fast in awakening, hence remember their dreams well. Persons who fall asleep slowly also awaken more slowly and are less able to remember their dreams well. In this latter group are the so-called non-dreamers. Hence this problem has little to do with a particular depth of sleep. Some psychoanalysts nonetheless hold the misguided opinion that the failure to recall dreams is the result of the painful, consciously suppressed content of dreams. This view is not supported by modern dream research, especially as fewer dreams having a painful content seem to occur than was asserted by psychoanalysts.

Sensations Occurring at Sleep Onset

Particular sensations that occur at the threshold between waking and sleeping do not belong in the realm of dreams. Typical transitional manifestations during this intermediate stage are extremely fleeting and vanish as soon as any attempt is made to register them consciously. As early as 1848, the French psychiatrist Maury was intensely concerned with experiences made during sleep onset, and he coined the term, hypnagogic, meaning "leading to sleep," to cover these sensations.

Sensory experiences without external stimuli

Sensations occurring during sleep onset consist of optical or acoustic sensory experiences that are not the result of any external stimulus. They include flashes of light, colored rings, waves, and other geometric figures, partly disfigured or fragmentary. Whole scenes with

47

action sequences similar to visions also occur. Acoustic phenomena include the perception of voices, hearing one's name called, or hearing entire fragments of conversation or music. The last-mentioned phenomena already belong, however, in the realm of complex hallucinations. One difference between hypnagogic hallucinations and dreams, which can usually be recalled, is their brevity. In addition, the person falling asleep remains an impartial observer of these phenomena. He does not experience himself as the acting person, as is frequently the case in dreams. Usually he can spontaneously distinguish between a dream and a hypnagogic hallucination. The person experiences himself as not yet sleeping, while in the course of a dream the person usually knows that he is sleeping or dreaming (Dittrich).

Dreams of falling   Another symptom occurring during sleep onset is a sudden, vigorous, jerky movement (myoclonus). It may be so strongly felt that it wakes the person up or flows right into typical dreams of falling. It is assumed to be caused by structures of the brain near the brain stem that are able to get past impulses from the cerebral cortex usually blocking them off. The result is the coordinated motor symptoms of the myoclonic jerk (Kugler).

Electrosleep

In the quest for safe methods of inducing sleep, experiments have also been made with electric current. However, before reporting on some experiences and thoughts about this problem, some references to various published materials on the topic are in place.

Electrohypnotherapy has been in use for several years. Its use was inspired in particular by Soviet scientists following the doctrines of Pavlow, who regarded sleep as a protective mechanism of the organism. The method could be only partially implemented, although indications

48

for its use were surprisingly extensive. Various initial reports concerning the use of this method were more or less optimistic. But voices were soon raised, cautioning against a too hasty utilization of electrosleep, particularly warning against electroanaesthesia since too little is known about the possible damage to cerebral tissue caused by electric shock therapy.

The same author, Mrs. Sommer, also reports on the results of experiments using electric shock therapy on animals. Preliminary tests confirmed that the indicated stimuli for electrohypnotherapy used on humans (in the realm of 20 to 30 hertz frequencies and voltages of 0.2 to 0.8 milliampere) did not induce sleep among experimental animals. She then describes the further course of investigation and ultimately the microscopic findings *Organic* concerning the anatomy of the brain. These illustrations *changes in* impressively show that the use of electrical stimuli *brain* definitely results in organic changes in the brain. *caused by* Therefore, it is evidently impossible to induce sleep *electrical* among humans through the aid of electrical current, *stimuli* because to do so would require the use of stimuli at a strength harmful to the brain. Lower voltages such as those used in animal experiments are not capable of inducing sleep in humans. As soon as the voltage is too high, or if it exceeds 13 milliampere, unpleasant sensations take place in the area of the sensory nerves of the face (trigeminus), especially in the forehead and back of the head.

Since the current ostensibly travels across the cranial bone, possible damage to the retinae of the eyes must be kept in mind. Under the safe limit of 13 milliampere, however, it is evidently never possible to induce sleep or a state resembling sleep.

Another author, Heppner, made similar statements critical of electrohypnotherapy by proving that only through external quiet and autosuggestions but not through electric shock therapy of the brain is it possible to induce a state resembling sleep.

49

Experiences in our clinic support his assertion. Many experiments clearly show that the effect is entirely psychological. As soon as the effect of the sleep machine abates, the same psychological patterns resume, as is the case in heterosuggestive treatment. Heterosuggestion differs from autosuggestive treatment and autogenic training, for example, in that an outsider makes the suggestion rather than the person carrying out the suggestion. Since the suggestion is made unintentionally and without the recipient's noticing the event or recognizing it as a suggestion, this method is also called *unintentional or unnoticed suggestion* (according to Stokvis and Pflanz).

To summarize, this means that so-called human electrohypnotherapy consists solely of light electric shock therapy of the brain. As long as it is administered within safe levels, it must remain ineffective for purposes of inducing sleep. For this reason, the term, electrohypno-therapy, should be completely avoided, since there is no such thing at present. Nor can sleep be induced by any of the electrical impulse machines constantly appearing on the market. Use of the term, electrohypno-therapy, does nothing but produce false hopes.

5. Sleep Disturbances —Causes and Consequences

Exogenous Disturbances in Falling Asleep

This kind of problem in sleeping is caused by a disturbing external stimulus or by a change in sleep rhythms or sleep habits.

Changes in sleep rhythm

Changes in rhythm occur, for example, in plane travel as a result of time changes. They also occur at work as a result of switching from the day to the night shift, on vacation due to the absence of the usual work schedule, or upon retirement. Paradoxically enough, difficulty in falling asleep as a result of unaccustomed exhaustion that upsets the organism's familiar rhythm also belongs in this category. A change of climate, an unfamiliar bedroom, new sensory impressions, acoustic stimuli such as strange sounds, or optical stimuli resulting from a room that cannot be darkened can become exogenous disturbing factors.

Difficulties in falling asleep resulting from such factors are considered to be physiological in origin if they again disappear soon among sleepers not usually troubled by

51

difficulty in sleeping—i.e., as soon as the body has
become accustomed to the new set of environmental
stimuli and has adjusted to the new rhythm or if the
environmental situation has changed. If normal sleep is
not resumed, however, and if the difficulty in sleeping
continues even after a longer period for adjustment, then
Psychic a real sleep disturbance is involved. This is termed a
reactions to psychically conditioned (psychoreactive) sleep distur-
external dis- bance, since the psychic reaction to the disturbance
turbances stimulus is the predominant factor.

Noise as a source of disturbance

Some sources of disturbance that clearly belong to
exogenous disturbance factors can subsequently lead to
psychically conditioned disturbances in falling asleep.
One of these is *noise.*

A disturbance from without can have the effect of an
arousal stimulus even to sound sleepers accustomed to
noise. The result is an exogenous disturbance to falling
asleep. If the person has become accustomed to the nois
and if the disturbance stimulus has become anonymous,
no longer seems to be very loud, and hence has lost its
disturbing effect, the person falls asleep despite the
noise. Sleep, as an active accomplishment by the
organism, takes place because it has been practiced
(conditioned) for a long time, i.e., it has been learned.

Subjective An additional factor in noise as a disturbance factor is
evaluation the subjective evaluation and the importance ascribed to
of the the source of the noise. The individual reaction prompte
source of by noise varies and can in time change. The disturbing
disturbance effect of noise is by no means in response to a
measurable magnitude or volume of sound. The disturbing effect depends far more on the individual evaluating
it. It also depends upon constitutional peculiarities and
upon the particular vegetative state of the organism. It
especially depends upon the mental attitude toward it

through which it gets the full measure of its disturbance value.

For example, a dog's barking may be registered as such a strong source of disturbance that it triggers a veritable chain of reactions ranging from fury to nervousness. It may be accompanied by heart palpitation and outbreaks of perspiration, physical pain, and ultimately violent aggression against the dog and its owner, but it can quite unsuspectedly vanish if one has come to know the dog owner as an appealing person and to be familiar with the dog's amusing, prankish characteristics. The barking then loses its disturbing quality, and one now knows or rather interprets when the dog is barking from pleasure or because children are playing and bothering him. Imperceptibly the concentration on the noise abates, separate phases of the noise are even ignored because of being freed from obsessively perceiving the noise as a disturbance.

Our au-
tonomic
nervous sys-
tem reacts
to noise

Apart from the responsiveness of the autonomic nervous system, which varies according to its condition, the vegetative reactions to noise are the only reactions that are dependent upon volume. While a healthy sleeper's consciousness can simply shut out a disturbance, the autonomic nervous system is by no means able to disregard "noise as a disturbance factor." It continues to register the irritation subliminally. Its reaction is expressed by a state similar to that of an awake, agitated person in whom the sympathetic nervous system, which functions as the trigger of the autonomic nervous system, dominates (ergotropic state of functioning). Sleep should be synonymous with calm and relaxation for the organism, though, and should be a trophotropic state of functioning.

A sound sleeper sleeps despite noise. However, the autonomic nervous system by no means gets the same recuperation from such sleep as it does from sleep in quiet surroundings. City planners and architects should know and keep this in mind.

Noise as a disturbance factor depends upon the *affective content* that the disturbance has for the sleeper. In other words, the affective content is the connection conditioned by feeling (emotion) between the stimulus and the recipient of the stimulus. It also depends upon the *informational content* of the noise.

Informational content of noises

Young mothers, for example, manifest a selective sensitivity to noise in what is called "the wet nurse's sleep." For a long period of time after delivery, they remain highly sensitive to even the smallest noises produced by the infant, while failing to register other low noises as an arousal stimulus. The same experience is confirmed by wartime experiences of soldiers who were able to sleep in the trenches through the thunderous roar of cannons but would become wide awake from the quietest ticking of the telegraph.

Attempt at muffling the sound

If the disturbances to falling asleep result from such external factors, there are several possibilities of help. The most immediate remedy, of course, is to reduce the noise, either through the use of double windows, heavily lined curtains, thick carpets, or by soundproofing the walls. Ear stoppers may also be helpful. Many people find them a problem, however, because they make one's own pulsebeat strongly audible. In addition, since they shut off acoustic contact with the world, they at the same time shut off sounds that one may wish to hear such as children crying or strange sounds in the house, and they make a conversation with one's spouse impossible.

Adopting a different emotional attitude

Still another measure should be to try to diminish the emotionally negative content of a noise disturbance. This can be accomplished through the use of reason— i.e., by attempting to place the disturbance in its proper context. Relaxation can also help, and it can be learned. Autogenic training, for example, or some other auto-hypnotic technique can aid in learning to relax and in reducing emotional stress. These techniques will be discussed in greater detail further on (see page 88). An advantage of such methods is that they can be used at any time. They enable one to let sounds simply pass through one without responding with tension and resistance, and they teach one how to diminish the affective response to the disturbance.

Snoring as a distur- bance

Under some circumstances, this method can provide the only possibility of coexistence between a snorer, who is otherwise an easy and even sleeper, and a non-snorer.

The reason for snoring is known. It evidently takes place mainly during the deep sleep phase—also possibly during REM sleep—through loss of basic muscle tension (muscle tone) in the musculature of the tongue and jaw. Snoring is most likely to occur if the sleeper is lying on his back, which causes the jaw to drop down and back and the tongue to slide back.

Sometimes the snorer even wakes himself up with his own snoring. In addition to the sound, which acts as an arousal stimulus, the snorer is awakened due to a lack of oxygen or shortness of breath. Snoring dependably wakes up the lightly sleeping partner and can even trigger a genuine wakefulness mechanism, since both persons become tense from the process of self-observation and expectation both of their own sleep and the sleep of the partner (mutually induced sleep disturbance). As a result, they are both impeded from falling asleep.

Still more grotesque (according to Finke and Schulte) is the process of "alternation"—i.e., partners alternate in disturbing each other's sleep. This occurs after the problem sleeper whose main obstacle to sleep was a snoring partner, has undergone successful therapy. Now cured of his difficulty in sleeping, he himself has started to snore and now keeps his partner awake.

Here, too, a problem that is mainly psychological creeps in. The snoring of another person is only felt to be disturbing if, apart from an allegedly abnormal sensitivity to noise and a low threshold of waking, the partner is in other respects felt to be "disburbing"—i.e., if tensions exist in other areas. The *affect* is the decisive factor in what is perceived as disturbing, so in many instances

Affect de- termines disturbance value

55

separate bedrooms are necessary.

But even the snoring sleeper can do something to help the situation. He should in any case lie on his side before falling asleep and should constantly drum into his consciousness, "I am lying on my side, I am going to continue lying on my side." With steady practice and in the course of time, this works like a well-learned resolution. It is effective and carries over into sleep. We will deal with these principles later in the section on autogenic training (page 88).

Condition of the bed

The importance of the condition of the bed is confirmed the moment one lies down on an unfamiliar hotel bed, when even a healthy sleeper can pass a sleepless night. Is there such a thing as an ideal bed? If so, what kind?

The best position for good circulation

There are two medical opinions on this topic. One is the orthopedic approach, which is concerned with the proper position of the spine. The other is more concerned with circulation, since heart patients, persons susceptible to circulatory disturbances, and older persons feel oppressed, anxious, and experience shortness of breath if

The best position for the spine

they lie in as flat a position as the spine requires. Their sleep may improve if a wedge-shaped bolster is used or if some other elevation is provided. On the other hand, persons having back pain and symptoms of slipped disks, who have difficulty in sleeping because they do not know which position permits them to be most free of pain, a firm, flat surface is recommended. Often a board placed under the mattress is an effective measure.

Temperature of the bedroom

There are similarly different requirements concerning room temperature and the condition of the bedcovers. Many people are dogmatic in their insistence on an ice-cold bedroom, others insist on wool blankets or prefer down quilts. The most important factor for sleep is plenty

56

of fresh air. Preferred methods of regulating room temperature by means of heat vary individually. Quite apart from the fact that a low temperature can serve as an arousal stimulus, persons who read before falling asleep or even for longer intervals of wakefulness during the night will probably not enjoy doing so in an ice-cold room. Not everyone likes to be covered up to the tip of the nose, which can also produce a feeling of oppression, difficulty in breathing, etc. A cool yet temperate room with sufficient fresh air, a warm light blanket, and a bed that suits the organism's physiological needs can in any case certainly help avoid difficulties in sleeping.

Sleep habits

It is important to drill good sleep habits. In particular, persons with sleep difficulties should repeat preparatory rituals every night. These include a fixed time for going to bed at the first sign of fatigue so the organism becomes accustomed to a regular hour for retiring. The regular habit of getting into a comfortable sleep position is also important. Most people prefer to lie on one particular side for falling asleep, and they frequently resume the position during the night. Sleep postures are attitudes that have been practiced for decades and have been drummed in through regular repetition. The mechanism that couples getting into the accustomed sleep position and then falling asleep is therefore important as a measure conducive to sleep. Especially when there is a change from familiar surroundings, as occurs for example while traveling, the practice of consistently retaining practiced sleep preparations aid in avoiding the threat of an exogenous disturbance to falling asleep and also helps overcome a new obstacle to falling asleep. The same time for going to bed, the same position, the same external sleep conditions (in the era of the car, many people even carry their own blankets), the same pre-bedtime habits such as reading, going for a walk, or hearing a little music are all devices for reinforcing and maintaining the sleep-wakefulness mechanism when it is subject to being undermined by external factors. If you are not immediately successful, just keep in mind that the body manages to get its necessary quantity of sleep and that little or no sleep for a night is not a danger to health. Rest is the most important thing. This statement, of critical importance in autogenic training, can be an important aid if remembered and really understood. The statement though, is important in two respects. For one thing, rest is the most important aspect of sleep; the second consideration is that if it has been possible to rest, the sleep pacemakers in the brain (pacemaker neurons) can exert their influence on the sleep-wakefulness mechanism and thereby set in motion the organism's active achievement, which is sleep.

The difficulty in adjusting to new surroundings is measurably increased if, as is the case on long plane trips, the biological clock also has to make an adjustment. If so, an adequate period of time should be allotted if at all possible to permit the organism to adjust gradually to the new local time.

Choice of reading material

As already mentioned, many people have the habit of reading before falling asleep, and it is repeatedly recommended as an aid in falling asleep. Well-intended suggestions of what to read range from the Bible to mystery stories. Mysteries, in fact, are praised as being especially effective as a soporific. And they probably are for normal sleepers, who anyway are not impeded by anything from falling asleep and are usually emotionally stable. Problem sleepers, however, should be careful in their choice of reading material. It should be something cheerful, contemplative, and preferably not exciting. For this reason, travelogues, short biographies, aphorisms, reading material that can easily be interrupted with the first wave of fatigue are particularly suitable. It should not be such exciting fare that the reader is driven to continue beyond the point of physiological readiness for

sleep, and it should not involve his interest to the point
that he cannot resist following the plot.

Psychoreactive Obstacles to Falling Asleep

Even the term for this form of sleep disturbance indicates
that it concerns difficulties in the psychic reaction to
events, experiences, or thoughts. Here, too, there are
nuances of what is "still normal," for even a healthy
sleeper can react to aggravating experiences by not
sleeping without at once being a problem sleeper.

Discrep-
ancy
between ex-
tent and
source of
the distur-
bance to
sleep

The line of demarcation to the abnormal is only
reached or even overstepped when the extent of sleep
disturbance no longer bears any relation to the cause and
when this situation starts to become a permanent
condition.

These sleep disturbances, as already mentioned briefly,
also have an element of predisposition, or of heredity.
Psychoreactive disturbances in falling asleep are often
found among persons who brood and mull over their own
moods and the moods of others to the point of becoming
depressed. These disturbances are also found among
persons having a tendency toward periodic depressive
states (cyclothymic personalities). Truly pathological
depressions (endogenous psychoses) that have come into
being independently and without perceptible external
cause are not at issue here; they are merely a
characteristic symptom.

Sleep disturbances among such cyclothymically dis-
posed persons originate in their tendency toward
brooding and self-criticism and in their being inclined
toward depressive reactions to experience (Schulte).
They are not able to shut things out or set aside the day's
experiences. They inwardly cling to all events. An added
difficulty is that they frequently reach their low point of

59

mood in the morning, similar to persons suffering from genuine depressive states. They therefore register their difficulties in sleeping particularly acutely in the morning, which accentuates their feeling of not having slept their full round.

The widespread discordant lifestyle of our modern world is characterized by insufficient physical exertion, overstimulation, the overrating of speed and accomplishment, and neglect of the realm of feeling. All these factors aggravate psychoreactive disturbances in

Socio-cultural factor

falling asleep. Relaxation, often sought only as a means toward increasing efficiency, takes its mental and physical toll also.

Although the precise consequences to sleep resulting from this sociocultural factor cannot be documented with figures, it is certainly not to be underrated.

Some tangible causes of this form of sleep disturbance are unfinished tasks, unsolved problems, or problems whose solution is unsatisfactory and therefore cannot be accepted, resulting in their being "worked on further" during the night. Particularly tenacious sleep difficulties are also caused by guilt feelings, real or seeming neglect, improprieties—in short, by a bad conscience. But a lack of sleep in this instance can have its positive aspects,

Productive aspects

because reflecting on such problems during the night can possibly lead to their temporary resolution. It is possible to come closer to the solution of many problems and to plan changes in attitude. The same holds for thinking things through, for which there is often during the day too little time, too little peace, and possibly a lack of distance from the problems. After a night of taking inventory and making important decisions, the person's inner security and clarity of judgment may make him able to cope with real tasks and problems. Efficiency on the following day is astonishingly little affected, perhaps even increased, and the subjective feeling of not having had sufficient sleep is remarkably slight.

Such "productive" encroachment on sleep, however,

60

is typically transitory. Such an encroachment only becomes a real sleep disturbance when the disproportion between cause and subsequent reaction steadily increases, when the process of reflecting during the night is not productive, or when it becomes fruitless repetitive brooding that is merely self-torture. If the psychoreactive disturbances to falling asleep were caused by unsolved problems and passing concerns, they can be eliminated by finding a solution to the conflict situation as quickly and as consciously as possible. In this case, the sleep disturbance can in fact be a kind of cleansing process. It is often worthwhile, instead of lying in bed and thinking about matters in the dark, to get up, turn on the light, and write down one's thoughts, which are often particularly concentrated and incisive at night. The consciousness of having written down the solution rather than having to retain it consciously brings relief, relaxation, and greater peace.

Reducing conflict situations

Writing down solutions to problems

Psychoreactive disturbances in falling asleep caused by very serious events such as sudden death, professional misfortune, dead end psychological or material situations constitute the few exceptions when temporarily taking sleeping pills is justified. However, if longer lasting conflicts possibly having their origin in the personality structure of the person are involved, sleeping pills are not a solution, and systematic psychotherapy must be sought.

Difficulty in Falling Back to Sleep

A disturbance in falling back to sleep again indicates that one fell asleep without too much difficulty, is soon awake again, and can no longer sleep. This kind of sleep disturbance is very disagreeable for two reasons— because waking up suddenly is often associated with a reaction of more or less strong anxiety, and because a

61

second attempt at falling asleep is usually more difficult than the first.

There have already been several references to the significant changes in reaction in the autonomic nervous system during the night. These changes are particularly strong during the first deep sleep phase. The depth of the deep sleep phase and the speed with which it is reached varies among individuals, and many persons only reach it once in the course of a night. Some of the changes that occur are changes in the blood supply to the brain, slowing-down of the rate of breathing, and the related electrolyte variations in the blood and the lowering of the blood pressure.

Persons having a tendency toward low blood pressure experience such sensations disagreeably upon awakening. The first deep sleep results in the significant lowering of the blood pressure, and this produces the feeling of anxiety. It begins with restlessness, tossing back and forth, the spiral-patterned worsening of the attempt to force sleep, making it increasingly difficult for the organism's own sleep mechanism to function.

Impeding drop in blood pressure

The leveling off of blood pressure that is too low was already discussed under the topic of sleep among the elderly, since fluctuations in blood pressure after the first deep sleep are especially pronounced among this group. But a cup of coffee drunk shortly before going to bed works as a paradox aid to sleep for all persons suffering from hypotension. Medications that generally improve circulation are also most helpful.

Overcoming nervousness by being quiet

The increasing nervousness and anxiety about not being able to fall back to sleep can be dealt with by various methods that facilitate relaxation and then lead to being able to fall asleep again. The first attempt in this direction is to remember that rest is of primary importance. In such instances, the precept of autogenic training, "sleep doesn't matter, but rest is important," can bring about a psychic reversal in which the person stops trying to force sleep and becomes more composed.

62

An opposite precept (a paradox intention) of trying not to sleep but to remain awake can also help. Additional recommendations are to try to achieve the greatest degree of physical relaxation and to lie on one's back, since lying on one side usually causes certain muscle groups to become tense. If this does not help, then a short air bath in the room (according to Tiegel) should be tried. This consists in walking back and forth in the room for two or three minutes without engaging in any activity such as reading, tidying up, gymnastics, or breathing exercises. Getting back into bed and snuggling into the comfortably warm spot under the covers in the familiar sleep position may then produce quiet and relaxation and possibly even sleep. The question of whether walking, which has a regulative and tonic effect on the circulatory system, or the comforting warmth of the bed promotes sleep is of secondary importance to the person able to get to sleep again by this method. The essential plus factor is that, having experienced success from one's own sensible behavior, one gradually gains new confidence in one's own ability to sleep.

Tiegel's air bath in the bedroom

Waking up Prematurely

Waking up prematurely is actually not a sleep distur-bance. More accurately, it is perceived as an exception and a disturbance if the person has wrong expectations or does not accept himself as a short sleeper. What is involved is hence a variation within the norm.

As with biological clocks and circadian rhythms discussed on page 24, some few people have a shorter-than-24-hour cycle. This shortening of the sleep-wakefulness mechanism is a form of instinct related, biologically determined behavior. It seems moreover to be coupled with a slightly hyperthymic personality type whose temperamental disposition is abnormally active, creative, and enterprising. The saying, "Morning hours

63

are golden hours," probably originated with someone inclined to be a short sleeper. In any event, the saying applies to a person having such a short sleep cycle.

The feeling of restoration in the morning depends, as already described, on the quality rather than on the duration of sleep—i.e., it depends upon the relation between the totality of the dream stages and other slee[p] Moreover, there is no immediate connection between t[he] day's activity and the need for sleep at night. Demands made on oneself during the day, a busy schedule, work done with verve and pleasure can even diminish the ne[ed] for sleep. Here, too, the initial psychic state determine[s] the restorative effect of the night. From the outset, the idea of not having slept enough is fundamentally *false*. [It] is false, because it refers to a non-existent *sleep norm* and to a *claim on sleep*. All that is accomplished by trying to meet such an absolute demand is to make life difficult without achieving anything.

The question of sleep before midnight belongs in this context.

At the end of the last century, a pedagogue by the name of Stoeckmann developed the idea of "natural sleep," meaning sleep before midnight. He enthusiastically promoted the idea that people who wanted to live healthy lives should, as a result of adjusting to sun time, go to bed early. Doing so would enable them to sleep as much as possible before midnight and would accord with a nature-given manner [of] living that consists of "going to bed with the birds."

If the person had slept enough, he should get up. eve[n] if it were only shortly after midnight. People who lived [in] this manner would soon notice that they can get along with substantially less sleep than other people and that the time gained, even if used long before the start of regular social activity, was a plus.

From various statements made by Stoeckmann, it ca[n] be concluded that he must have been a person with a short circadian cycle and that he simply made a credo o[f]

64

of his early waking pattern. The same tendency applies to quite a number of thought associations made in one narrow area of thinking where the method used is to tone down or to emphasize ideas, depending upon how they fit into the theory. Many intellectual novelties are actually credos. Stoeckmann's sun-time thoughts may have been mixed up with health improvement ideas, as was the case with Kneipp, Schroth, and many others.

The danger of feeling under pressure of time in falling asleep

Even though Stoeckmann's views could not be verified, they nonetheless contain some laudable psycho-hygienic aspects, especially for the present era. Anyone who goes to bed before midnight has a better chance of starting the day well rested. By going to bed early, he is no longer under the pressure of time in having to fall asleep quickly. He can calmly look forward to the many hours of sleep ahead, which is in itself relaxing because it eliminates the compulsion toward success.

Unlike people in the average household, he does not need to subject himself to the evening TV, which is emotionally and probably even physically burdensome. TV is frequently associated with a heightened danger of intoxication (risk of poisons) as a result of smoking and drinking while watching it. For example, if an actor on TV lights a cirgarette simply because the script has not provided any instruction on how to fill a gap, millions of viewers imitate the gesture without even realizing it. It is no different with reaching for a drink. It should be kept in mind also that dogs avoid TV and move away from it. They hear the overtones, and although humans do not hear them, who is to say that their autonomic nervous system does not register them as an excitation?

Anyone who follows Stoeckmann's precepts and goes to bed early is not confronted with any of these dangers. But to some extent he lives in an anti-social manner, since civilized living also includes evening social life. It would surely be preferable to plan more active, social evenings rather than being compelled to submit uncritically to passive social communication. Stoeckmann's

Planning an active evening

65

ideal life style of sleeping before midnight can then be valid for us today without our having to become apostles of health.

People who are early risers, either because they go to bed with the birds in accordance with Stoeckmann's principles or because they, as hyperthymic personality types, are bursting with morning energy, usually do not suffer from their habit of getting up early. At best, the only ones who suffer from their waking habits are those in the immediate vicinity who are perforce swept up into fervid activity.

Functional Sleep Disturbance

Clinical findings and subjective assessment

Functional sleep disturbance (or functional hyposomnia) is the most frequent and therefore the most important form of deviation from healthy sleep. This term applies to a group of sleep disturbances in which the disturbance is functional—i.e., is not the result of an exogenous (resulting from external causes) or of an endogenous (having its origin in the body) illness. The term *functional* hence expresses something about the function, meaning that the structure of the function is disturbed without directly making any statement about the cause (etiology). Frequently the interplay of various regulatory mechanisms is disturbed at the same time without the reason being known.

Definition of functional sleep disturbance

Neurologically the combined symptoms of the disturbance of function that subsequently leads to functional sleep disturbance probably consists in the disturbed course of the synchronic and asynchronic sleep phases. Instead of the normal cyclical change, a rapid oscillation (phase change) occurs between different deep sleeping and waking periods where there is altogether too little deep sleep (Baust).

66

These findings explain why so many persons suffering from functional sleep disturbances have the feeling of not having slept at all, even when they did objectively sleep. The impossibility of the individual's precise assessment often makes diagnosis significantly more difficult.

The difficulty already mentioned of a person's judging himself to be still awake or already asleep was documented by Baust (1967) in very clear observations made concerning sleep experiments made in a laboratory: "Many subjects assert upon awakening from the stage of sleep onset or from light sleep that they were wide awake and had been thinking about something. Consequently, in the stages of light sleep it is impossible to make precise statements about the degree of wakefulness.

"Similarly, a group of subjects asserted upon awakening from dream stages that they had been wide awake. Dreams, too, are often interpreted as thoughts experienced while awake. The explanation for a patient's assertion of utter sleeplessness is consequently the result of more light sleep stages or the false assessment of dream phases."

Clinical and neurophysiological evidence has strengthened my view that the subjective feeling, "I have slept," that every normal sleeper has upon awakening is evidently coupled with the periodic alternation between synchronic and asynchronic sleep phases. If this alternation is missing, as for example in the constant oscillation between light and deep sleep of the person suffering from functional sleep disturbance, the subjective feeling of having slept is also absent. This again shows the close connection between physical feeling and psychic assessment—i.e., the somatopsychic aspect from which sleep and especially functional sleep disturbance must be considered.

The course of such functional sleep disturbances is definitely chronic. Severe forms of sleep disturbances often begin as early as in the third decade of life, or between age 20 and 30, and then manifest a slow and

67

constant increase. Only rarely is the pattern of development one of periods of worsening, alternating with periods of remission.

Waiting for sleep

Functional problem sleeper's fear of the bed

External events are often blamed for difficulty in sleeping until the affected person concludes that sleep disturbance persists even after gradual elimination of the obstacle to sleep and even after the many attempts to obtain treatment have also proved unsuccessful. Such persons frequently develop a real anxiety about the bed. Even during the day the thought of going to bed produces an attack of anxiety. As a consequence, they develop a tendency to go to bed at an increasingly later hour, which only aggravates their difficulty in sleeping. Many, if not all, persons suffering from difficulty in sleeping tensely wait for sleep at night, completely forgetting that sleep cannot be forced. As early as 1905, Dubois wrote, "Sleep is like a dove. If you quietly extend your hand, it will light; if you reach for it, it will fly away."

Falling asleep cannot be forced

The practice of going to bed at a later and later hour and the increased desperation in waiting for sleep, of wanting to force sleep to come, can only aggravate functional sleep disturbance and make the initial psychic state a real and insurmountable barrier to falling asleep.

Reaching for the sleeping pills

The linkage of wrong attitude and wrong reaction, a real vicious circle, which should in this instance be understood quite literally as a steady increase in pain, climaxes in reaching for the sleeping pill. At this stage, however, the pill can hardly be effective except in significant dosage. And the problem sleeper who, at least subjectively, has spent many sleepless nights, has only the one dominating wish to be able to sleep, and wants the pill to have the effect of a sledgehammer and to have the effect of bringing about sleep at any price. So he

68

no longer considers whether a sleeping pill is healthy or has side effects if it will only help. He is then neither particularly careful with the dosage, nor does he hesitate to have recourse to alcohol. Since the combination of sleeping pills and alcohol is particularly dangerous, it must be treated in detail in a separate section (page 99).

An underdose of sleeping pills has as disastrous an effect as too large a dose. Underdosage occurs mainly among persons who take advice from other problem sleepers and even try out their sleeping pills either because their own medically prescribed pills no longer help or because they, despite being afraid of unfamiliar medication, start doctoring themselves without medical counsel. So they start with too low a dosage to be effective in aiding them to fall asleep or to make them less nervous and tense. Then, after having waited too long, they increase the dosage of sleeping pills by timidly taking another half-tablet, which again is insufficient to induce sleep. In this manner, intake and reduction of medication can almost be balanced out without ever achieving the therapeutic level that results in sleep, and the sufferer can "creep up on" two or more sleeping pills in the course of a night without ever falling asleep or eliminating his steadily increasing tension.

The feeling of exhaustion resulting from not having slept off too large a dose of sleeping pills is particularly acute on the following morning and lasts well into the day. It is certainly more unhealthy and strenuous than a sleepless night. Consequently it is necessary at this point to warn emphatically against the dangers of dilettantically

prescribing sleeping pills for oneself. Every medication works in its own way, every person reacts differently to one and the same medication, depending upon his physical and psychic state at the time of taking it, and therefore requires dosage specifically appropriate to him and his state of health.

Those who have suffered from sleep disturbances

69

for several years often convey the impression of physical exhaustion and look pale and tired. Mentally, though, they are usually easily irritated and tense and often lack initiative, verve, and pleasure in planning their lives. These characteristics are still more pronounced among chronic users of sleeping pills. Such problem sleepers often manifest other vegetative symptoms such as nocturnal sweating, anxiety states, and an abnormally fast heartbeat, and frequently have a tendency toward depressive states. The typical pattern of their vacillation in mood shows them to be at their lowest point in the morning after having slept poorly and waked up too early.

Hangover effect of soporifics

Thus functionally disturbed sleepers reveal both types of personality. Some are the subdepressive cyclothymic type who can find no end to brooding, who pile up problems instead of eliminating them, who wall themselves in with their problems almost to the point of being crushed by them, whose initial response to any issue is negative and problematic, and who are unable to sleep because of their self-torturing thought processes. And then there is the other, hyperthymic personality type who is unable to sleep because of the excitement of pleasant anticipation, creative drive, and an abundance of ideas. While both types may experience the same degree of difficulty in sleeping, in the last analysis they differ from one another in their opposite evaluation of a situation based on their respective dispositions. The subdepressive cyclothymic type can feel ill from the awareness of having a sleep disturbance, while the other personality type experiences no suffering in connection with being a short sleeper and therefore comes to terms with the condition without any physical ill-effects.

Subdepressive personality structures

The last dream phase before waking can also be decisive for the feeling of having slept well or poorly. This is true even though the person may be unable to recall the dream and regardless of the quality of sleep periods preceding the last dream phase.

Nocturnal anxiety

Vacillations in mood because of the darkness

What makes lying awake subjectively so disagreeable to many persons suffering from functional sleep disturbance, in addition to experiencing concomitant vegetative symptoms, is the experience of night and especially darkness as an additional negative factor. This reaction is not restricted to persons having cyclothymic dispostions. Many persons who react to the night in this manner are by day unusually active, cheerful, and well-adjusted, with no traces of suffering from problems in sleeping or of experiencing night terrors and despondency. Evidently there is a special form of nocturnal depression among persons whose mood varies greatly with light. On sunny days they are irrepressible and in a mood of feeling they can embrace the world, while they almost become depressive during long periods of gray and fog. Paradoxically or typically, they sleep better during the bright, short summer nights than during the long winter nights. This tendency concurs with observations made in Scandinavian countries, especially Lapland, where sleep disturbances are more prevalent and evidently more severe than in comparable countries at other latitudes. Where there is too much interruption in the circadian periodicity and in the normal sleep-wakefulness rhythm, light as an arousal stimulus and darkness as an inducement to sleep therefore seem capable of producing psychic imbalance.

What can be done, though, about such functional sleep disturbances? How is it possible to cope with them without becoming hopelessly dependent on sleeping pills? Let us remember man's biological clock and think of sleep as an instinct-related event that can be learned.

Social and biological rhythm

If light had for the human sleep-wakefulness mechanism the same imperative meaning of being an arousal stimulus as it does for birds, or if darkness were similarly an imperative command to sleep, therapy would be no

71

problem. Since this is not the case, however, and since our social rhythm takes precedence over our biological rhythm, we ourselves must assume control over our attitude toward sleep. We choose the time for falling asleep, after all. We have learned to "control" our biological need for sleep. We remain awake until we permit fatigue to take over. In other words, we are prepared to give in to the organism's demand for sleep so the pacemaker neurons can act on the centers regulating sleep and produce sleep.

Social life as the time-marker

How strongly social life as a time-marker can influence the biological rhythm can be seen to a large extent by observing house pets that have even adjusted to human rhythm.

The learned alienation from the biological command to sleep poses no special problem to the normal sleeper who is able to readjust his sleep-waking pattern relatively quickly and can almost spontaneously fall asleep while standing. But the functional problem sleeper can and must combat such alienation. This can be done by restoring the importance of the biological sleep rhythm and by responding to the natural need for sleep, which will result in an improved ability to sleep.

Choosing the time for falling asleep

That is easier said than done, however, since the effort involves permitting one's own need for sleep to triumph over the life rhythm of the immediate environment, and it includes an attempt to live at odds with social demands. Such an attempt initially makes it difficult to live with other people who can go to bed any time they choose. It is by no means necessary to adopt Stoeckmann's ideal of sleeping before midnight or of going to bed with the birds. What is needed is to accept the necessity of really giving in and going to bed at the first feeling of fatigue.

Establishing the time for falling asleep according to biological need

The condition for success with this measure is to secure the cooperation and understanding of one's companions similar to the manner in which consideration is shown someone about to take an exam or to a nursing mother. What is primarily meant is that the family's

72

understanding must be sought by explaining the situation to them, because the sleep regimen will necessitate some changes in family living. For example, if a mother of half-grown children whose activities increasingly take place in the evening deviates from the family rhythm, or if a wife whose husband comes home relatively late in the evenings adopts for herself a rhythm of dining at 5:00 p.m. and going to bed at 9:00 p.m., an interruption in family life occurs. Since, however, only a limited period of time is needed for a person to learn to sleep again, most families can cope with the change.

Inducing fatigue

In addition to noticing and giving in to natural, periodic signs of fatigue and wakefulness, it is necessary to induce this alternation between recuperation and fatigue, activity and relaxation, between work during the day and rest at night. Of primary importance is an external, noticeable break between day and night. This does not apply to lying down and snoozing for two hours in front of the TV before going to bed. It does apply, though, to remaining active until the beginning of the first sign of feeling tired and can be achieved by engaging in some light activity, by an evening walk, or by a stimulating visit with friends.

Establishing a break between day and night

The evening meal must also be eaten early, perhaps between 5:00 and 6:00, so that enough time remains before going to bed. If possible, functional problem sleepers should really get a workout during the day. Work in the garden is good therapy for this purpose. And they should remain active until evening. Under certain circumstances, afternoon rest should be curtailed, because a one-hour nap is subtracted from sleep during the night and must be counted, too.

Planning the evening

In order to be able to make the psychological switch from day to night, sufficient time must be allowed for a

73

Let the day
taper off

really meaningful evening. This necessitates letting the day come to an end. Setting aside problems and concerns is an ability that can be practiced and ultimately learned, and is necessary for getting into a good mood and gaining some perspective on matters. Usually it is far more helpful to read or to engage in an interesting conversation than to look at TV. Unlike the passive receptivity involved in watching TV, reading, for example, can bring contentment through the activity of one's own thoughts. By reading it is possible to push aside the day's events by one's own positive initiative. TV tends to gloss over the day's events, and often leaves behind a frustrating emptiness that can promote depressive moods.

Give in to
the first sign
of fatigue

Once one has started to notice the first sign of fatigue, one can confirm its regular manifestation at about the same time. If one then gives in to it regularly, one learns a new reaction of making an association between time and going to sleep. Certainly the worst thing one can do is to constantly postpone the time for going to bed because of anxiety about being unable to sleep. It is important to establish the act of going to bed as an expression of biological rhythm.

The necessity of going to bed early was well formulated by Tiegel, "The crucial factor in any treatment of sleep disturbances is regard for the natural, systematically occurring signs of getting tired and of waking up." Elsewhere he said, "The problem sleeper should continue the day's activity as usual and go to bed as soon as he notices the beginning of a pleasant feeling of fatigue and of a desire to go to bed. He must heed the natural sign of fatigue. All of us encounter it daily, though we disregard it or try to eliminate it by whatever artificial means, either because it disturbs us while we are at the theater, listening to music, or are at a lecture, or because it comes as a nuisance while we are doing some evening chore." Elsewhere he states specifically, "If a sick person is suffering from nervous sleep disturbance, the first measure to be prescribed is that the person make it possible to lie down to go to sleep at the start of the *first* sign of getting tired, regardless of any obstacle provided by family or surroundings. At the *first* sign of waking up after a few hours of refreshing sleep, the person should get out of bed and start the day's activity.''

Get up as soon as you wake up

So here, too, it is seen that people are encouraged to notice and respond to their biological clocks. Maybe it is really worthwhile once again to notice light as a time-marker of the circadian periodicity of man's biological clock. Then we can relearn what we have unlearned, which is how to sleep. As already stated, the healthy sleeper can afford to unlearn registering light signals, but those with functional disturbances cannot.

I know of several persons suffering from severe functional disturbance who resorted to trying to regulate their sleep-waking cycle by becoming attuned to their biological clocks. By using all available aids already described in part, they were successful after a period of time, and were gradually again able to fit in within reasonable limits with the average family rhythm.

Functional sleep disturbances can be inherited

For the benefit of the next generation, let me repeat: functional sleep disturbances accumulate within the family, and clearly manifest inheritable genetic traits. For this reason, children particularly threatened by this possibility should be trained to being oriented toward their biological clocks. This means they should be put to bed at the proper time. It is worthwhile sparing them the possibility of later becoming problem sleepers, and it will certainly minimize the possibility.

Probably the experience of missing sleep is subjectively the strongest factor among functional problem sleepers, especially if they compare themselves daily with healthy sleepers in their vicinity who tend to describe their own sleep in such glowing terms as excellent, wonderfully refreshing, and splendid.

But just as it is necessary to live with personal handicaps in other areas, it is necessary to realize that it

75

is senseless to run amok inwardly against a disposition toward sleep disturbance. Perhaps knowing that one must live with a sleep disturbance helps somewhat; knowing that one can live with it has helped many to get over the difficulty. There are many things in life toward which we should not have a quarrelsome attitude. This statement can apply to many areas of life—to one's own profession, to one's legal status, to the feeling of inferiority, and many other things, not to mention real physical handicaps. One condition it does apply to is functional hyposomnia. The quotation from Hoelderlin may not be to everyone's liking, but since it was made by Hoelderlin, who knew what he was talking about, it carries great weight and should be included here: "Stomp on your suffering, and you will stand taller!"

If the functional problem sleeper does not want to quarrel for years or forever with his suffering, he cannot avoid a positive attitude toward the findings concerning lack of sleep. For this reason, it would be gratifying if many readers could take this advice to heart. It definitely contributes toward gaining some distance or toward at least becoming indifferent to the disturbance.

This important reorientation can be further supported by all the measures already discussed—by following Tiegel's recommendation of taking an air bath in the bedroom and by concentrating on rest if it proves impossible to fall asleep again after having slept for a short period of time.

I myself always make a practice of reading both before falling asleep and upon waking up, and I recommend this practice to all functional problem sleepers. What seems to me more important than the acceptance or rejection of this suggestion is the question of whether the person was already always accustomed to reading to fall asleep. If so, it is a dependable method of slowly turning off the wakefulness mechanism. The necessity of focusing one's eyes while reading produces the need to rest them by changing their direction, and can lead to a kind of trance

76

state similar to what occurs in step-by-step active hypnosis to be discussed later.

The functional problem sleeper who masters these thoughts has mainly learned to adopt an *emotionally neutral attitude* toward the feeling of a lack of sleep. As a result, he is less depressed and dull upon awakening, a state that is probably mainly a result of negative experiences during a night perceived as sleepless. If the negative experiences abate as a result of having come to terms with the state, this too has a positive effect on the person's mood the following morning.

Waking up—getting up

Many insomniacs feel that they wake up "too early" or "prematurely," and they then frequently postpone really waking up. The countermeasure is to get up promptly. The inner command to be given by both healthy and problem sleepers is "wake up and get up!" And the command must be responded to immediately, since there is evidently a "hangover" even without sleeping pills, which are known to produce hangovers, ostensibly a psychic condition that has something to do with lingering in an intermediate state between waking and sleeping.

Don't doze off after waking up in the morning

The unfavorable effects of dozing on into the morning can even be observed in children, so the habit of getting up immediately after awakening must be practiced from an early age. Here, too, the importance of the learning process in connection with regulating the sleep-wakefulness mechanism is apparent.

The means of refreshing oneself after awakening and getting up are such an essential part of body hygiene that no comment is needed here.

If a functional problem sleeper wakes up some time before the start of the usual day's activities, he should get up, dress sensibly, and start the day in a comfortably heated room. I know quite a number of intellectually creative problem sleepers who get up and start work as

77

soon as they wake. The most extreme example is one who gets up at 2:00 a.m. These very early morning hours are extremely productive for many people, however, and the quiet helps them to concentrate. Persons engaged in other activities can find many possibilities for using these early morning hours.

Many problem sleepers have the feeling in the morning of not having slept *enough*. After all that has been stated thus far, it is so obvious that little need be added. But the contrast between the healthy and problem sleeper will certainly be less if all the suggestions made are followed. The possibilities of gradually building up a program of self-help have been repeatedly pointed out, and anyone wishing to adopt these aids should do so step by step. Success is the certain result.

6. Factors that Disturb Sleep

Snoring

Practice formula resolutions

Snoring, as already discussed in the context of psychoreactive disturbances in falling asleep (page 55), doubtlessly also belongs in this chapter, because its disturbing effect cannot be denied. Since it has already been so extensively treated, however, the reader should just be reminded again that snoring can best be dealt with through autogenic training, using formula resolutions. The person should lie down on his side some time before going to sleep and repeatedly resolve, "I am lying on my side, and I am going to continue to lie on my side." With consistent practice, this will in time have an effect even during sleep.

Tooth Grinding

The habit of tooth grinding during sleep, bruxism, is disturbing to the person doing it and to others in the vicinity. For some unknown reason, with few exceptions the habit only occurs among girls and women. Readings measuring the rhythmic activity of the chewing muscles during sleep confirm the presence of the habit. The

79

practice occurs in all phases of sleep and is most frequen
in the intermediate and deep stages of synchronic sleep.
Since the chewing muscles involved in tooth grinding ar
very strong, noctural grinding is by no means harmless.
can result in the significant wearing away of the teeth an

Tooth and
jaw
prophylaxis

eventually in deformation of the jawbones. For this
reason, anyone having this habit should consult a dentis
immediately. It is most important that he see about the
possibility of learning autogenic training, which is quite
effective in dealing with this problem. It can even be
learned by older children, who are likely to be motivate
to do so if they suffer from the habit.

Sleep-Talking

Sleep-talking is a form of intensive dreaming, and
therefore occurs in most instances during the asynchron
sleep phases. It occurs more frequently among children
and young people than among adults. It has no particula
significance and therefore requires no further discussion

Sleep-Walking

Sleep-walking, or somnambulism, is not actually a sleep
disturbance. Even though it occurs during sleep, it is an
abnormal form of being awake, as revealed by telemetri
readings of the brain. Sleep-walking evidently involves
special kind of waking state that can neither be called
waking nor sleeping. This form of sleep could be termec

Split state
of con-
sciousness

a split state of consciousness (dissociated) in which ther
is motor wakefulness and psychic sleeping. The coordir
tion of the motor functions, or movement, and the
processing of optical sensory stimuli occur during
sleep-walking beyond the state of consciousness (subco
tical). Consciousness of being wide awake is not at all
present.

80

Sleep-walkers often develop astonishing motor abilities that can more readily be explained by the abnormal waking state than by the sleeping state. They are able to find their way through pieces of furniture placed close to each other, they can walk on top of narrow walls, and even climb around rooftops. Many a sleep-walker has in fact even leaped out of a window and awakened only upon landing on the street with a broken leg. Seashore describes a student who got up from bed, dressed, walked to a river about a half mile away, undressed, took a bath, got dressed again, went home, carefully folded his clothes and put them on a chair, and got back into bed to continue sleeping. When he awakened the next morning, he could not remember anything at all about his nocturnal outing.

Occurs mainly among children and young people

Sleep-walkers have their eyes wide open; they look straight ahead, though they seem to look into emptiness; they take no notice whatever of their surroundings, and their movements are stiff and awkward. Sleep-walking occurs mainly among children and young people. It is more rare among adults, but may possibly occur with some frequency among persons who in other respects have sudden or unmotivated fluctuations in consciousness. For example, if people do not remember in the morning what took place during the night although they were awakened for a brief period of time, it can indicate a heightened tendency toward this form of psycho-vegetative instability. The cause is not known.

Since there is no real possibility of treating such conditions as sleep-walking, all that can be done is not to permit persons inclined toward sleep-walking to sleep alone without being watched over. Some precautions should be taken while they sleep.

A state of *sleep drunkenness* that occurs among persons who awaken with difficulty actually involves a postponed awakening. During the minutes or perhaps only seconds of clouded consciousness coupled with disorientation that may lead to senseless, usually harmless acts, the person is already capable of motor activity. Only in very rare instances can such a condition become dangerous—for example, if the persons attempts to catch alleged burglars or attackers while still in the state of sleep drunkenness. When the person wakes up completely, he experiences total amnesia and can remember nothing about what happened. Some care must be taken to avoid provoking them, because sometimes the person may feign the condition, possibly for purposes of concealment. Such persons should simply be permitted a little more time to come back to reality. The state does not last very long, and quiet surroundings help terminate it.

Night Terrors

Waking up with a fright (*pavor nocturnus*), usually screaming and crying, is related to sleep-walking. It only occurs among children and is clearly coupled with anxiety. Many children remain in bed, others wander around in confusion like somnambulists. If the child is very anxious, it often seeks protection and refuge with the mother. Spontaneous awakening does occur, but mostly the children go back to sleep, and they can then be awakened only with difficulty. In rare instances, it can *Extreme* be shown that the state is related to exciting events of the *anxiety* previous day. More often, though, anxiety and more serious problems that can only be reached and treated by psychotherapy are involved. Strictness and "psychic toughening" are of no help whatsoever with this problem, and in severe cases the possibility of psychotherapeutic treatment should be considered. A dim light in the room of a child inclined toward night terrors can be helpful by making it possible for him to find his way about.

Rhythmic Tossing Back and Forth of the Head

The rhythmic tossing of the head back and forth at night (*jactatio capitis*) involves a stereotypical rhythmic head movement among children. The movement, evidently pleasurable, usually starts just before falling asleep and continues even in half-sleep. It can become a habit, and although it doesn't disturb the child, it frequently disturb others in the vicinity. It can remain constant over long periods of time, then usually ceases of its own accord. The habit is best broken by being ignored as much as possible.

Nocturnal Bedwetting

10%-15% of all children are bedwetters

Nocturnal bedwetting (*enuresis nocturna*) as a disturbance is so important that it must be particularly stressed in this passage. It is extremely widespread; 10% to 15% of all children suffer from it. Often the condition is wrongly diagnosed and is not properly understood by doctors. Certainly the sympton of bedwetting cannot be overlooked. What is meant, though, by wrong medical diagnosis of the condition is the failure to distinguish accurately between the two forms of bedwetting. The cause of each is fundamentally different and therefore requires a different therapy. Anyone who does not know this will moreover wonder why this phenomenon accompanying a child's sleep is considered a sleep disturbance. In fact, it must be regarded as a real symptom of a sleep disturbance.

Secondary bedwetting as a regression to earlier childhood behavior

What is meant, however, is not secondary bedwetting that occurs among children who were dry a moment before the incident and who already have mastered at around age two the complicated task of controlling the. bodily functions. The cause of this form of wetting can b prompted by a withdrawal of love resulting from the arrival of a new sibling or as a protest reaction against a

83

decisive change of surroundings such as being placed in an institution or clinic. Such trauma causes the child to regress to earlier behavioral patterns (regressive), consequently losing the already learned capability of reacting to the stimulus of a full bladder by getting up and emptying it. This form of bedwetting is doubtlessly a problem in behavioral psychology and has nothing to do with sleep disturbance.

But the problem of *primary nocturnal bedwetting* is another matter. Children having this disturbance sleep extremely soundly. It is impossible to awaken them, and if one attempts to place them on the pot, they simply go limp. The same thing happens when one puts them to bed. Even when they start to wake up, they are unable to use their muscles, because the muscles are too lacking in tone. If, despite everything, they have urinated and are put back to bed, on the following morning they can remember nothing about the incident. Bedwetting typically is repeated several times in the course of a night. And this happens despite having emptied the bladder in the interval and despite having limited the intake of fluid. Often they may not have had liquid since noon of the previous day.

The sleep disturbance underlying this behavior consists in extended and extremely deep states of sleep. The vesical sphincter seems to relax during these periods of sleep, and the other muscles that control the emptying of the bladder contract. This usually occurs before a dream stage, because as a rule no dream experiences are reported upon awakening.

Another striking characteristic of the disorder is that evidently children with a cyclothymic personality structure are most inclined to have this form of sleep disturbance, which again shows what a close connection exists between this disposition and sleep problems. On the other hand, this correlation provides the opportunity, especially with these children, of controlling bedwetting through the use of suitable medication, as is also done in

84

treating endogenous depressions.

Any attempt to counter this form of bedwetting through limiting fluid intake is utterly wrong, because bedwetting two or three times during the night is not the result of a specific quantity of fluid. It is caused by the endogenous production of fluid, which is unaffected by the intake of a specific quantity of fluid. Among these children, the condition is often the result of a reversed circadian periodicity. While normally the production of fluid controlled by the mid-brain is strong during the day and slight at night, the process is reversed in primary enuresis. Therefore the practice of witholding fluid after noon on the preceding day of its occurrence represents a complete failure to recognize the essence of this disturbance. Many children are subjected to the incredible hardship of being denied fluid without the slightest chance of bringing about improvement.

Among retarded children

Still another constitutional factor to be mentioned among such children is a tendency toward delayed development. It is also one of the reasons that this disturbance vanishes of itself at such a decisive moment in maturation as puberty. Among girls this if often the age at which menstruation begins.

From all of the above, it is clear why this form of bedwetting involves a real sleep disturbance. And once this is realized, it is no longer necessary to subject children to the discomfort of withholding fluids for long periods or of wrongly emphasizing psychic problems. The bedwetter can, however, be given psychological support by stressing positive events associated with the disturbance—for example, by keeping a monthly or quarterly chart for recording nights that were *free of such symptoms*. The opposite effect is achieved by charts that record the negative events for the purpose of being able to show the doctor "when it happened again." If a family feels shame about such a sympton of illness among one of its members, the result is true psychic oppression of the child.

85

7. Therapeutic Methods

Psychotherapy for Sleep Disturbances

Psychotherapy is to be understood here as a treatment using psychic means. Defined in this manner, it includes many of the recommendations made by psychotherapy both in the broad and in the narrow sense. The recommendations nonetheless belong more in the area of psychohygiene intended to impede the worsening of already existent disturbances.

If the question is asked of why so little is known about psychotherapeutic methods of treatment of sleep disturbances, it should be understood that in practical terms the only question concerns psychoreactive disturbances in falling asleep and functional hyposomnia. There is reason to suspect, especially concerning functional hyposomnia, that an analytic treatment as practiced by psychotherapy would not reveal much. The reason for the ineffectiveness of psychotherapy is that these functional sleep disturbances do not involve an abnormal psychic (neurotic) development; they involve tendencies deeply rooted in biological development.

These psychic tendencies are direct consequences of this physical condition. In less frequent instances, they are indirect consequences of the physical condition. They are therefore psychological signs of illness in a narrower sense. They are psychic reactions or manifestations of a psychic inability to cope with a bodily disfunction— namely, of the inability to sleep. If such psychopathological conditions are involved, analytic psychotherapy has hardly any relevance to the condition and little promise of success. The use of psychotherapy among functional hyposomniacs has been so fruitless that it has hardly been worthwhile to publish anything about such treatment.

Psychotherapy exists, however, in forms other than analytic therapy and includes many other kinds of treatment in addition to those methods already described here in some detail. These methods may either be the normative pragmatic technique of a concrete, treatment-oriented form of therapy or may be objective
psychotherapy, which is considered supportive. I prefer to call these methods active-autohypnotic procedures, because this term characterizes both the technique and the goal.

The designation, "active," as used here means that the method emphasizes concentration for achieving relaxation. Initially this is done by achieving muscle relaxation as a step toward reaching other psychic changes best described as a self-induced trance that is very similar to a state achieved through hypnosis and autohypnosis. Autogenic training, as one of the most important methods of these autohypnotic procedures already mentioned so frequently, will be described in the next section.

Autogenic Training: Learning to Be Quiet

This method of treatment was developed toward the end of the twenties and first summarized in book form by J. H. Schultz in 1932. The extensive description of autogenic training to be made in this section should not, however, tempt anyone to begin the exercises without a doctor's guidance, since occasionally complications can result from study without instruction from a specialist. Experience shows that problem sleepers have particular

Difficulty in relaxing

difficulty in relaxing, being limber, and in letting themselves go. If this were not the case, they would probably have no difficulty in sleeping. For this reason, though, they most of all need an introduction, explanation, and guidance about how autogenic training works. Left to themselves to learn the methods, they would fail, would no longer place any confidence in the technique, and that would definitely be a regrettable loss. They would have lost a chance to acquire a significant aid in better coping with their difficulties. The problem sleeper should consult a doctor skilled in using the method and learn it in private or in group sessions. He will learn the basic principles of autogenic training, or of "psychotherapeutic basic exercises," a term to be encountered again in discussing the methods of graduated active hypnosis.

Exerting an influence on yourself by concentration

There are several steps in autogenous training, a technique of exerting influence on the self through concentration that leads to the achievement of a trance state resembling a hypnotic state. After tapering off into a quiet state, concentration is used to achieve muscle relaxation. This results in altogether diminishing basic muscle tension (muscle tone). Relaxation spreads through one arm and gradually through the whole body. Since this process is neurophysiological in origin, it is felt and experienced as weight. Instructions to the person learning the method require him to imagine this weight by using passive concentration. After some practice, all that is required to bring about muscle relaxation (generalized hypotonia) that spreads through the entire body is to imagine "rest—weight," and almost instantly he will experience *rest and weight*.

The next exercise is directed toward regulating the

89

Regulating the blood vessels

blood vessels in the arms and legs and then in the whole body. A real, measurable widening of the vessels does occur, even among persons just starting to learn muscle relaxation. Several examinations enabled me to prove that this does take place, although it usually is only noticed when the concentration is focused on experiencing warmth. Here, too, the trainee starts by imagining a feeling of warmth in one or on both arms until he is keenly able to experience warmth in the extremities and even in the whole body. Therefore he should concentrate on imagining "quiet—weight—warmth."

The state achieved by these means was termed basic psychotherapeutic exercise by E. Kretschmer, who developed the method of step-by-step active hypnosis (1946). The directions of the two methods diverge beyond this point. After other more advanced training is mastered, the continuation of autogenic training leads to meditation. The continuation of self-hypnosis, however, leads directly to a hypnotic state or to a state resembling hypnosis and is achieved through practice in keeping the eyes motionless (prolonged fixation) for an extended period of time.

Redirecting breathing

In contrast, test subjects continuing basic autogenic training, after attaining the feeling of warmth and weight spreading through the entire body, next practice changing their breathing by imagining the somewhat strange but particularly effective phrase, "it breathes me," or "it breathes in me." This does not explain the idea that breathing is primarily a passive event. Once the student has had his attention called to his breathing, he is impeded from inadvertently forcing his breathing or from overbreathing (hyperventilating). He learns to observe his breathing, which produces a generalized effect of relaxation and automatically switches over to passive breathing.

It should be mentioned in this context that all oriental forms of meditation achieve an autohypnotic state by means of regulating the breathing. Juxtaposed to the

exercise in inhibiting breathing that occurs in several
forms of yoga is the "regulation of breathing" used in
these autohypnotic methods ". . . until the breathing
becomes excellent and joyous," as Buddha expressed it.

Regulating
the
heartbeat

The second exercise directed toward the functioning of
an organ concerns the heartbeat. The resolution to be
concentrated on is "heart is beating quietly and
vigorously" or "heart is beating quietly and evenly."
Through these exercises, it is literally possible to feel the
heartbeat slowing down and to show a slight drop in
blood pressure.

The next step is to concentrate on regulating the blood
vessels in the abdominal cavity. This is done by using
concentration to try to reach the nerve plexus responsible
for the degree of constriction among the abdominal blood
vessels. This nerve plexus has long been termed solar

Regulating
the vessels
in the ab-
ominal re-
gion

plexus or plexus solaris, hence the command, or better
yet the inner imagining should be "solar plexus flowing
warm." An improved blood supply to the abdominal
organs takes place as a result of concentration.

In the last exercise at the elementary level of
autogenic training, the head is stressed as the center
that guides the body by concentrating on "forehead
cool" or "forehead pleasantly cool." In contrast to all
other exercises, all of which aim at relaxation and
vegetative change, the last exercise deals with a primarily
psychological phenomenon. Problem sleepers are emphatically recommended, however, to omit this last exercise
in their attempt at achieving relaxation through the aid of
autogenic training, as it can easily be registered as an
arousal stimulus.

91

Graduated Active Hypnosis: Learning To Shut Things Out

Basic psycho-therapeutic exercise

In graduated hypnosis, training is only given in feeling the weight and warmth that spread through the whole body and arms and legs. The more advanced exercises concentrating on breathing, the heart exercise, and the regulation of the blood vessels in the adominal regions–i.e., the so-called visceral exercises (from viscera, the intestines)—are omitted and are supplemented instead medically supervised training in fixing the gaze, which leads to an autohypnotic trance state.

Which of these two methods, autogenic training or step-by-step active hypnosis, is preferable for use in correcting functional sleep disturbances? There is no generally applicable answer to this question. Since I ha been more involved in graduated hypnosis, I can think more valid arguments for this method. By limiting the exercises to the generalized weight-warmth experience or the basic psychotherapeutic exercises, more time is gained for focusing on concentration, which after all w the reason for learning the exercises. The exercises to omitted are those for the heart, breathing, the abdomin vessels, and the exercise in registering the feeling of coolness in the forehead.

Practicing individual goal con-cepts

Beyond mastery of the basic exercises, both methods. autogenic training and graduated hypnosis, have some points in common. Exercise programs for both techniques include the use of individual goal concepts that must be systematically worked at. These guiding principles are expressed as slogans in the case of activ hypnosis, and the resolutions in autogenic training are expressed as formula phrases.

Both the slogans and the formula phrases used by th two techniques should as a rule consist of two parts. I first necessary to strive for as much indifference as possible to the disturbance; and, secondly, the goal to attained must be stated.

But what use is to be made of these methods by the functional problem sleeper in particular? What aids do they offer him? Before it is possible to explain the answer, it is first necessary to know more about the origin and nature of such meditative methods as autogenic training and graduated hypnosis.

The inner attitude acquired through meditation was worked out on the basis of knowledge about the Buddhist trance, a special form of oriental meditation. The next-to-the-last state before achieving the ultimate Buddhist trance state of nirvana is the state of "sancta indifferentia," or the state of holy indifference. Since these methods of achieving a trance state enable persons to reach a very deep psychic level of feeling and emotion, they produce a beneficial resonance suppression in the feeling reactions (affective resonance suppression). This means that approaching stimuli are experienced less strongly, they can be met with greater indifference, and the emotional or feeling connections to the disturbing symptom are impeded. Similarly, all external stimuli are so weakened by a heightened stimulus threshold of nerves leading to the center (centripetal connections) that they are transmitted to consciousness only with difficulty or not at all. As a result, the feeling connection to the disturbances and the sensitivity to stimuli of the centripetal connections are changed or diminished in the autohypnotic state.

An indifferent attitude attained by these means is useful in the treatment of sleep disturbances. The first part of the formula phrase learned in autogenic training is "sleep is never important." Once this precept has been learned and firmly fixed in the imagination, it can be shorted to "sleep unimportant." As already mentioned, this results in an intensification, which means coming to terms with one's own disposition to sleep little or to sleep in short intervals, coming to terms with not having a positive or pleasant experience in sleeping, and in neutralizing the feeling of being unable to achieve

esonance ppression f the feeling reactions

93

restorative sleep.

The second step in these resolutions or slogans should be directed toward attitude, which is more decisive than sleep, because if one has the right attitude, sleep can spontaneously occur. The second step therefore involves the concept of rest, and the exercise in concentration is "sleep is of no concern; rest is important!" The conception (imagining) of rest should to some extent positively strengthen the feeling of indifference to the disturbance. In this manner, the feeling of neutralizing the sleep disturbance and of positively strengthening the feeling of indifference toward sleep sensibly compliment each other.

Positive reinforce- ment of the idea of rest

These methods were described in such detail in order to show how fundamentally helpful they are to problem sleepers and to encourage them to learn to relax with the help of a doctor. Once they have mastered these methods, they can continue to practice them alone.

Practice in fixating the eyes

The necessary exercise in fixing one's gaze already learned in graduated hypnosis after having mastered the basic psychotherapeutic exercise must always be practiced only under medical supervision. Only after complete mastery of this technique and with the doctor's approval may one continue to practice it alone. Since the most important exercises must anyway be done in the dark, the gaze is not directed toward an object. It suffices simply to look into the darkness without fixing one's eyes on anything; or it is possible to practice looking from within with closed eyes at one's own forehead. This resembles one aspect of instruction given by Schultz for making the transition in autogenic training from the elementary to the advanced level. I think, though, that the most important thing for problem sleepers to do is look quietly into the darkness for a period of time. After a while, the eyes will close by themselves. The further steps in the idea to be concentrated on, "rest— weight—warmth" and "sleep unimportant—rest important," will then lead to the goal of beneficial relaxation.

Problem sleepers should also know they can never attain such deep autohypnotic trance states through autogenic training or step-by-step active hypnosis as can some other persons practicing these techniques. They cannot do so because of their compulsive natures and their inner difficulty of permitting themselves to let go. Persons so constituted, even if not specifically suffering from sleep disturbances, only achieve a more superficial trance. They should not be disappointed about it, however. What they should rather do is to realize the obligation to take to heart all the other suggestions made. There are many roads to success!

Paradox in-
tention
Brief reference has already been made elsewhere to the "paradox intention," which states that persons suffering from pronounced fears or phobias should strive for what they fear. For example, persons afraid of blushing should diligently and expressly try to blush. According to my observations of problem sleepers, such a paradox intention makes sense when there is a strong fear of sleep or anxiety about the night. It is then possible, in various ways as described above, to try out a paradox intention such as making an effort to keep one's eyes open and to look into the darkness with the intention of remaining awake.

But if the person does not have an expressed fear of sleep, this should not be attempted, since it makes tense persons still more compulsive, and that would achieve nothing.

In their efforts to cure themselves, insomniacs may gratefully sieze upon such suggestions made by well-meaning friends as "count backwards from 1,000," "count sheep," or "think of nothing at all," but these attempts lead to nothing. Precisely how "think of nothing" is to be done is not explained further. Even yogis require years of training before being able to focus their thinking to the extent that consciousness is excluded and total amnesia occurs, which represent the last steps in "thinking of nothing at all."

95

Unsuccessful attempts to think of nothing are more likely to make problem sleepers still more restless. This applies not only to them but perhaps to all persons who strive for something without being able to attain it.

Apart from this last negative example, however, the other methods already discussed for achieving sleep or rest agree in principle on the necessity of distracting the problem sleeper from his difficulty. Thinking should be directed toward a certain set of ideas and should be kept there. It leads to an important aspect of the autohypnotic state, which is the narrowing of the field of consciousness in order to stimulate other aspects. It leads specifically to a lowered state of consciousness.

And which psychic state is attained by these techniques? A *partial sleep,* which can then change into real sleep. That is the goal in mind, and that is the chance!

Progressing from being partially asleep to being completely asleep

8. Burdens and Apparent Aids to Sleep

Sleep and Stress

The concept of stress is now often used in too broad a sense. As with other psychiatric terminology, care should be taken against using familiar terms too comprehensively, because their meaning gets lost and becomes diffuse, which is what has happened with many terms such as hysteria, psychopathia, neurosis, etc.

For this reason, I would like in particular to define psychic stress as follows: psychic stress should be understood as a mental burden that (1) goes beyond a general burden and (2) is specific to the individual person through whom it becomes pathogenic or becomes an illness.

Defined in a narrow sense, stress is a *relative* and *circumscribed* excessive burden.

Stress varies with the individual

In this context, *relative* means that not every person is susceptible or vulnerable to the same stress. *Circumscribed* expresses the thought that in many areas the personality is not receptive to stress but is receptive to stress according to its individuality in narrowly limited areas. For example, persons with a tendency toward vacillations in mood—the cyclothymic personality structure already described (see page 70)—are especially vulnerable in situations involving change. What is involved may be a change in residence, a move to a new

97

location, or a change among people familiar to them. Schizoid personalities, on the other hand, are especially vulnerable to religious problems and to problems involving sexual drive, and these problems can become stressful for them. Persons with partial delayed development (in Krestchmer's terminology, partially retarded personalities) are vulnerable to demands made on them from the area of demands corresponding to their age but which, for these persons suffering from delayed development occur too early.

Persons with heightened, nervous irritability or, to express it differently, with a heightened psychovegetative lability, are more easily vulnerable and more receptive to stress from stimuli that increase this nervous irritability. Such stimuli include many originating in our technological society, noise, increased work tempo, irregularities in the rhythm of day and night that place too great demands on their sleep-wakefulness mechanism, and still many others.

Stress chains

Events, life situations, or activities accordingly can lead to such specific overstress which, although in and of itself not a burden, can become a burden in reference to the individual by exceeding the quantity of excessive demand, hence become stress. The origin of a whole chain of stresses often cannot easily be perceived, since the affected person only makes the last link in the chain responsible for his overstrain. In addition, factors not accepted as stress factors are suppressed and accumulate. The person then suffers from what appears to be excessive demand in one area with which he is in reality perfectly able to cope. The true origin of this situation, the discrepancy between burden and receptivity to burden, is either not recognized or is not accepted. If a sleep disturbance is the final result of such an individual chain of burdens, then in this instance understandably sleeping pills are senseless, since they only suppress a symptom without approaching the cause of the stress situation.

98

But it is possible in this instance—and this should be clearly recognized—that the sleep disturbance can have a decisively beneficial effect. It can be used for reflecting on one's own situation, the different factors that led to the stress situation, to think about one's attitude toward the situation, and peacefully and calmly to get a broad perspective on one's life, to sort out one's thoughts, and to work on clearing up and eliminating problems.

Recognizing the physiological necessity of a minimum amount of sleep, one or two sleepless nights can be consciously used nonetheless for writing down certain more far-reaching perceptions. Having something on paper can have a real unburdening effect. A burdensome thought can be placed in a neutral context, even if only a piece of paper. Even the positive attitude toward clearing up one's own problems and the activity involved in doing it can have a beneficial effect by blocking the feeling of being delivered up to a situation.

Alcohol and Sleep

Alcohol has become accepted by many persons as a help in case of need. The range of recommendations for using alcohol is as broad as the choice of drinks is abundant. Since alcohol ranks with drugs in being dangerous, a fact glossed over for a long time by the publicity given to the use of drugs by the younger generation, I want to convey a few thoughts about the topic. Two things must be made clear: the effect of alcohol on the central nervous system and the possibility of dependence. The topic of dependence resulting from the use of sleeping pills requires discussion as well. The concept of addiction must be dealt with, as the number of addicts, especially of persons addicted to alcohol in Western industrial countries is extremely high and steadily increasing.

Considering the great number of alcoholics in our society, alcohol as a "sleeping aid" or as a means of inducing sleep must be subjected to careful examination.

Alcohol affects the central nervous system

Alcohol attacks the brain—i.e., the central nervous system. But it also affects the vascular system, the autonomic nervous system, and is a particular burden on the liver, which has the task of breaking it down. The poison in alcohol permanently damages the liver cells, causing fatty degeneration and contraction that result in cirrhosis of the liver.

Since the liver cells to some extent "learn" to lay in a supply of the necessary ferments for breaking down poisonous substances—in this instance, alcohol, but similarly for other substances such as sleeping pills containing barbituric acids—the quantity of alcohol or the dosage of sleeping pills must be increased to achieve the desired effect. This changing interrelation between substance and organism is termed "tolerance." It is extremely high among opiates (morphium and related substances), regardless of whether they are in their natural form or are synthetically produced. It is approximately equally high for alcohol and preparations containing barbituric acids, so the danger of a resulting physical dependence (in the sense of addiction) is great.

Liver cells learn to adjust to poisons

Tolerance is accordingly explained by the liver's ability as a detoxification organ to break down all substances having a poisonous effect and its special capacity for being able to adapt its cells to certain poisons. The liver is therefore able to break down these poisons with increasing speed. In addition, since alcohol, like almost all substances affecting the central nervous system (psychotropic drugs) can affect one and the same person differently at different times and under different circumstances, alcohol is without exception to be ruled out as a sleeping aid. Other psychotropic substances should also be subject to strict medical control and should be administered only for very limited periods of time. Even the slight amount of hops contained in many alcoholic drinks makes this attitude imperative. A tiring effect that would correspond to a real "sleep dosage" is greater than the dosage that can be tolerated, and is therefore in the realm of the toxic. The danger of addiction resulting from constant usage by unstable persons, in addition to damaging the liver, is unavoidable. Conspicuous misuse also results in damage to the brain cells.

The concept of addiction

As should be clear from the above, "addiction" is understood to be a physical dependence on a substance, the quantity of which must constantly be increased in order to achieve the same effect. Severe mental and psychic consequences result from the omission of or withdrawal from the substance, and these are termed withdrawal symptoms.

Psychic dependence

Soporifics also conceal, as will be described (on page 102), the danger of physical dependence or at least of psychic dependence on the medication. Just as a smoker, in whom there is no developed physical dependence, cannot imagine a TV evening without a cigarette, so it is with the person accustomed to alcohol. In particular, every person dependent upon soporifics knows that one of the first steps in preparing for a holiday trip is to obtain a prescription for an adequate supply of the familiar sleep medication that he depends on. Although the absence of the tablets would not cause any physical withdrawal symptoms, it would spoil the holiday.

Heightened effect of alcohol and soporifics

Since, as already mentioned, physiologically the target attacked by alcohol is basically the same as for soporifics, the effect is increased if both drugs are taken simultaneously. Persons dependent upon soporifics or persons having an abnormal alcohol intake increase the potency by taking both at the same time. In this context, barbituric acids have a particularly strong effect since, like alcohol, they work extremely quickly. The resulting condition is particularly dangerous to the nervous system. Car drivers should always be aware that the combination of alcohol with soporifics or tranquilizers often has an increased effect that lasts well into the day.

101

Sleep Medication and Sleep

There is really no such thing as a medicinal therapy against sleep disturbances, since sleeping pills only eliminate lying awake but not the sleep disturbance. The sleep disturbance can, in fact, be aggravated by medication, which in turn can lead to an additional dependence upon sleeping pills. This expresses with utter clarity the sober fact that sleeping pills only doctor around the symptom without in the slightest changing the cause. And, in addition, it does so with means detrimental to the organism and its ability to function.

The difficulty of precisely judging the effect of soporifics on the brain consists in the fact that several activating and deactivating systems are responsible for directing the sleep-wakefulness mechanism. Nonetheless, the reaction to the most important medications by separate areas of the central nervous system has been investigated in experiments on animals through the insertion of microelectrodes into the brain. Results show that a centrally situated part of the brain, the reticular system, which is among the most important structures directing the sleep-wakefulness mechanism, undergoes changes from sedatives or hypnotics such as soporifics containing barbituric acids and from tranquilizers such as Valium, Librium, and many others. The changes caused by all these medications do not occur in this form in physiological sleep. Electrical activity in the brain and clinical manifestations in the central nervous system that occur during sleep induced through medication only resemble those occurring during natural sleep, while differing in essential respects.

Changes in the physiological sleep pattern

The most important question for us in this context concerns the effect of medications on the separate *sleep phases*. Their effect on the asynchronic sleep phase (REM sleep) interests us most of all, for it also seems to be the more important of the two sleep phases. But before explaining this in greater detail, it is first necessary to discuss the various groups of medication under consideration.

Sedatives or Hypnotics

Barbiturates

The soporific most familiar to the medical layperson is the group called barbiturates, which are varying combinations of barbituric acids (barbituric acid derivatives). They have been used in medicine since 1903. Since that time, 2,500 barbituric acid combinations have become known. Approximately 50 are on the market, and ten or twelve are in frequent use today. They are known under the trade names Veronal, Seconal, Dalmene, Evipan (hexobarbital), Luminal, and many other designations. Since some of them can in fact induce sleep rather quickly, as for example Evipan, they can also be used as light anaesthetics, which is not generally true of sedatives.

tispasmodic effect

The effect of barbiturates on the central nervous system ranges from having a slight soothing influence to inducing sleep, coma, and even death from sufficient overdosage. Barbiturates affect numerous biological functions, the central nervous system, the heart muscle, skeletal muscles, and the smooth musculature of the blood vessels and digestive tract. Phenobarbital (brand name "Luminal") is so effective in relieving cramps that it is one of the most important medications used in treating spasms. Habituation and addiction occur frequently as a result of using barbiturates and can be a serious problem.

Many hypnotics have a sedative (tranquilizing) effect and influence the central nervous system in a manner similar to that of the barbiturates. Although they are completely different in their composition and pharmacological properties, they usually have the same side effects and disadvantages as the barbiturates.

Potassium bromide

The oldest and structurally the simplest of these drugs is potassium bromide, which is contained even today in

103

numerous headache preparations and sleep medications available without prescription. It is important to know, however, that it is very slowly excreted by the kidneys, and longer period of regular use can result in an absolutely poisonous accumulation (toxic accumulation) that produces numbness, diminished ability to think and observe, and emotional instability.

Chloral hydrate — Chloral hydrate, which also belongs in this group, became famous on the crime circuit, where it was known as "knockout drops." When a few drops were added to alcohol, it has a very rapid and intensive effect, and it was used to incapacitate prospective robbery victims.

Dorides — Doride for a long time was mainly considered a competitor of the barbiturates. It was assumed not to have the same side effects and in particular was not considered addictive. In the meantime, this assumption proved false. Its chemical structure strongly resembles thalidomide that gained an infamous reputation. All of these medications have primarily been investigated from the standpoint of their effectiveness on the central nervous system, and the procedures used in investigating chromosome breaks and genetic mutations are still too recent to permit a comprehensive summary.

Meprobamate — Another hypnotic that is effective as a sedative is meprobamate. This substance also has primarily a tranquilizing effect. Because of its ability to diminish anxiety, irritation, and tensions, it also has a sleep-inducing effect. Medications containing meprobamate were long overrated, because people were glad to have any substance that had a tranquilizing effect without containing barbiturates. Meprobamate was nonetheless classified by the Food and Drug Administration as a drug comparable to barbiturates in its potential for misuse. The ruling was contested in court by the manufacturer, which continued to designate it a "minor tranquilizer." Meprobamate is contained in Milltown, Equanile, and several other preparations.

Numerous medications produced by several different

104

firms belong to the group classified as tranquilizers. The effective substance contained in all of them—such as Valium, diazepam, and others, as well as the well-known Librium—is oxyzepam.

The Two Forms of Paradox Sleep

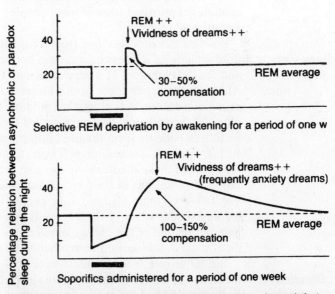

This diagram compares the sleep setback (sudden change) that occurs during paradox (asynochronic) sleep after the administration c barbiturates with the setback effect following REM deprivation causec by selective arousal. As can be observed, the periods of the REM phase ascend and are extended after the dose of barbiturates. The vividness of dreams, often of a negative kind, is also extended. The duration of this abnormal reaction is, in comparison with relative REM deprivation, significantly longer, as an average REM is attained only later. (Based on a curve by Oswald, i.)

105

All of these drugs affect the central nervous system, but in far more different ways than the barbiturates. They affect the cerebral cortex and the *formatio reticularis,* which was already mentioned in connection with the attempt to localize the sleep-wakefulness mechanism in the brain. Because they also affect the thalamus and the hypothalamus, centrally located brain structures important in the feeling reactions, the ramifications of their use are extensive. In addition to lessening our motor capacities, or active muscle movements, they diminish emotional responsiveness and bring about a change of mood tending toward primary euphoria—i.e., an immediately improved state of mind coupled by diminished anxiety and tension.

Danger of dependence on medication

Possible dangers resulting from frequent and continued used include an influence on certain hormone controls and the development of a dependence on the medication. Although the dependence in this instance is primarily psychic in nature, it is altogether possible to speak of a physical dependence, having observed how difficult it can be to free patients from the use of diazepam preparations such as Valium, Tranxilium or Tavor, to mention only a few. Use of these medications can also produce extreme physical symptoms in the form of disturbances in the vegetative system. Also not to be overlooked is the increased adaptation of the liver cells as evidence of habituation and of the change in tolerance already mentioned in connection with other drugs.

Dream deprivation resulting from barbiturates

But let us return to the question of how these medications influence the separate sleep phases, especially the REM phase that is so important and, among other functions, is responsible for dreaming. Barbiturates seem to suppress the asynchronic sleep periods, resulting in time in a genuine "dream debt" or "REM debt." Consequently, both the number of rapid eye movements and the total duration of the REM phases seem to be shortened, and the quality of sleep is noticeably affected. Tranquilizers, on the other hand, if tests made thus far

106

can be believed, do not seem to shorten the total duration of REM phases; therefore the sleep pattern yielded remains natural. To be sure, tranquilizers do not actually bring about sleep. What they do is rather to make way for sleep by calming the emotions and reducing motor activity. However, when patients discontinue taking these preparations, especially if they have taken them over a period of time, they have the same complaints as patients leaving off preparations containing barbituric acids. They are disturbed in particular for several nights by continuous, intensified dreaming, or by making up for the "dream debt."

The other important question concerning the use of medications to influence sleep is whether it is wise permanently to suppress affective disturbances, which should provide motivation toward psychic reorientation or maturation (Holm). Should there not preferably be an attempt to interpret period of short sleep and longer waking periods as a protective measure of the organism? Or even regard such periods as a psychic process of cleansing and reorientation that is needed by the body? Seen from this point of view, the suppression of these self-regulating processes can be harmful to the organism, and the attempt to hurl the body into sleep is perhaps physiologically unsound. What mainly happens, though, is that the organism simultaneously forgets how to bring about sleep as an active accomplishment without the aid of medication. In any case, the impression is conveyed that through continued use of soporifics, the switching function in the sleep-wakefulness mechanism is, at least hypothetically, lamed. The organism is definitely deprived of its activity in bringing about sleep. Larger dosage of sleep medication changes the normal sleep pattern in the direction of "general anaesthesia." (Finke and Schulte)

After sleep medication is discontinued, the total length of time spent sleeping is shortened for several nights. Through the aid of sleeping pills, sleep is also at the same

Waking periods as a protective mechanism of the organism

The organism forgets how to sleep

107

time borrowed, so this debt must be paid back also. It is seen, however, that among functional problem sleepers who continually use sleep medication, a real debt has been incurred that can never be quite paid back. The decision to discontinue use of the medication is always followed by a period of increased sleep disturbance until the organism has been paid back its sleep debt and relearned its own function.

Sleep deprivation resulting from medications

There is a clear parallel between sleep induced by soporifics and by anaesthesia, but the description of such sleep bears no resemblance to healthy sleep. The sleep onset experiences that occur without the use of medication are mainly characterized by a relatively long intermediate period between waking and sleeping during which the limbs become heavy, and the arms and legs become warmer. The eyelids also become heavy, so that if the person is reading before falling asleep, it is hardly possible to finish the line, and it then becomes impossible to start the next line. Gradually the letters become blurred, and the gradual inability of the eyes to focus resembles a state achieved in graduated hypnosis (see page 92).

Relation between sleep induced by soporifics and by anaesthetics

This intermediate stage is marked by several typical psychic changes. It becomes increasingly difficult to maintain a train of thought, and a thought process called "free association," which is characteristic of sleep onset occurs. At the beginning of such a thought process, the person has reached a certain point in thinking about a topic, and then suddenly finds himself thinking about something else without having any notion of how he came to the new idea. Only after consciously thinking about it can the connecting points of the thought process be traced. The closer one gets to sleep, however, the greater the missing links or leaps from the beginning of one thought to another. A vivid description of this phenomenon is included in a Taoist meditation, "The thoughts are like monkeys on the trees. They leap from one branch to the other." In the course of coming closer

Free associative thinking

to falling asleep, the thoughts vanish, and finally a state of "rhythmically repeating unconsciousness," which is the historic definition of sleep, is reached.

Sleep onset experiences are short-ened

These intermediate stages of sleep onset are frequently quite protracted. They are drastically shortened, however, in sleep induced by soporifics. Anyone who has ever been given an anaesthetic may similarly recall that the stages of falling asleep occur so rapidly that it is impossible to experience them. Because of this parallel to sleep induced by anaesthetics, the term, "anaesthetic sleep," occurs to me whenever I think of sleep induced by soporifics. Sleep induced by an anaesthetic is actually a phenomenon of extinction, or of slight death, which is how sleep was formerly regarded. In any case, the kind of sleep brought on by sleep medication bears no resemblance to sleep as an active accomplishment by the organism.

The danger of dependence on medications resulting from taking soporifics over a longer period of time has already been referred to several times. The layman must recognize this danger in order to take responsibility for seeking other avenues of help. Formerly there was talk of "habituation" or "addiction." Since the concept of addiction if ambiguous, however, the World Health Organization has been influential in supporting the use of

Drug de-pendence

a broader term, "drug dependence," which still includes dependence on medication. The following concepts were then derived from the comprehensive designation of drug dependence: physical dependence, which corresponds to addiction, and psychic dependence, which means habituation. There is not a clear line of demarcation between the two conditions. As already described, both can occur, so reference is made to specific types of dependence, and types of dependence are then described in terms of specific drugs or medications.

Barbiturates are doubtlessly more dangerous than benzodiazepine and meprobamates. Therefore anyone taking them and especially any doctor prescribing them for extended periods of time should consider the risk of dependence on barbiturates. Sedatives not containing barbituric acid also lead to a dependence on medication, as already described. And although such dependence is largely psychic, a physical dependence in the realm of the autonomic nervous system is entirely possible. For this reason, every problem sleeper having any contact with these substances should take care that the ingestion of such substances is only temporary. Unfortunately, however, the opposite usually occurs. Since the effect of benzodiazepines (Valium, Librium, Tavor, and many other medications) is registered as especially pleasurable and also because they produce a slightly elevated (euphoric) mood, patients repeatedly ask their doctors to renew their prescriptions. For his part, the doctor is glad that his patients are happy, consequently easily inclined to renew the prescriptions. In addition, although many doctors regard benzodiazepine as harmless and even discount the danger of dependence, American textbooks on psychiatry emphatically call attention to this danger and even specify the preparations most frequently prescribed.

Failure of sleep cures
In closing, some observations concerning the problem of *sleep cures,* since chronic problem sleepers repeatedly request its inclusion. There is practically never occasion for such therapy, and there are many arguments against it. If prescribing soporifics to problem sleepers is problematic for reasons already mentioned, the same is still more true concerning sleep cures. If sleep cures are undertaken either in response to a patient's strong insistence or because a doctor inexperienced in treating problem sleepers believes they may be effective in breaking the vicious circle, such efforts will be dependably futile. In comparison with other

Danger of overdosage
persons, these patients require a much higher dosage of tranquilizing medications, which increases the danger of reaching the harmful toxic level. What is sooner achieved than sleep is a delirious state characterized by confusion

110

and a clouded consciousness. In addition, it is necessary to keep in mind the resulting dream deprivation that must be made up during a subsequent phase of shortened sleep periods. The patient's response is disappointment, because in effect he is back at the start of his problem.

9. Your Own Sleep Analysis

You have probably bought this book, because you yourself sleep poorly, because this problem at least interests you, or because you know someone suffering from difficulty in sleeping and want to help.

It is only possible to help oneself and others if one knows whether one has a real sleep disturbance, what it is about, and what can be done about it. We have tried to show that inability to sleep is a problem that can be avoided. Admittedly, however, it is a problem requiring our insight, learning abilities, and an energetic commitment to combat it.

The necessity of keeping a record of one's own sleep and at the same time making notes about one's habits and disposition is a means of becoming informed about oneself. It is also an important step toward therapy.

Categorical judgments Almost all problem sleepers express their difficulty in sleeping in categorical terms. They say, for example, "I didn't sleep last night at all." "I didn't close my eyes until early morning." "I heard the clock strike every quarter of an hour." Because of such estimates, they then say, "I am completely done in. I am tired and depressed. I am completely exhausted. I can't go on."

It is possible for a person to have such a strong feeling of being sick that the sickness assumes a value, hence effectively carries the same weight as a real organic

113

*Conscious-
ness
of sleep dis-
turbance
impedes
sleep*

illness. In addition, the feeling or the consciousness of not being able to sleep can become so decisive that the person can no longer sleep, and the awareness of the difficulty can impede the ability to sleep. The imprecise descriptions of seemingly sleepless nights and their consequences show how strongly consciousness of a lack of sleep and the resulting exhaustion is anchored in the realm of feeling.

The reason for making a written record of your own sleep regimen, for placing it in relation to your habits, and analyzing it is primarily for the purpose of establishing whether there is a direct relation between the amount of time slept and the feeling of recuperation, which factors possibly affect sleep, how events of the day affect the quality of sleep, how the time for going to bed works out, whether and how the presence of the partner affects sleep, and to draw all the conclusions from the data. The conclusions may possibly include accepting the fact that you are by nature a short sleeper. Or the conclusions may show that you had become accustomed to going to bed at the wrong time; because your optimal time for falling asleep is either earlier or later. Perhaps to your surprise you will discover that you can sleep alone more undisturbed, that you should eat much earlier in the evening, that you should go for a walk in the evening, or that you should read instead of watching TV. So the task is to find out what helps your ability to sleep, what has unconsciously disturbed you or even kept you from sleeping until now. Only after you know the nature of your specific sleep problem, which was previously registered as an unconscious feeling of being unable to sleep, is it worthwhile drawing up a sleep plan specifically for you and for your needs. The goal of such a project is to exclude all factors that disturb you personally, to create your optimal sleep conditions, to eliminate your preconceived ideas about yourself and how poorly you sleep, to assume a positive attitude toward the whole problem, thereby making it possible to

114

initiate a learning process and to establish your own appropriate sleep pattern.

When you are certain about the factors affecting you personally, write down a list of suggestions that you can really implement:

Finding out which sleep habits work best for you

• Eliminate to the greatest extent possible all such external disturbances as noise, light, wrong temperature, wrong bed. In some instances, it may be necessary to have your own bedroom. Discuss all these matters with your family, because each member of the family should assist you to the best of his ability in your efforts to learn to sleep again.

• Adhere to the practice of going to bed at the hour most conducive to your being able to sleep, even if your social life must be neglected for a while.

• Try by means of autogenic training to assume an indifferent attitude toward periods during the night when you are not asleep, toward seeming to fall asleep too late and use the opportunity to try to learn to rest.

• Use interruptions of sleep sensibly by reading, by air baths in the bedroom, by writing down pertinent ideas that may assist you in solving your problems, and go ahead and get up if you realize that your tendency is simply to wake up early.

• Don't count up the number of hours you slept. Enjoy the days when you feel fresh and well. You will realize that these by no means necessarily follow nights when you slept an unusually long time. Perhaps you will soon notice that it is possible to get along with relatively little sleep during periods of some especially pleasurable activity. The fixed idea of equating a lot of sleep with efficiency and a small amount of sleep with exhaustion will vanish by such factual evidence to the contrary.

• Understand that sleeping pills provide no solution to your difficulties and don't take them.

• Trust the experience that the organism gets its minimal quota of sleep required for maintaining its functions.

• Try to assign sleep an increasingly lower value on the

scale of things you consider important.

• Remember that sleep is an instinct-related event that can be changed by learning processes and that it is an active achievement of the organism.

• Keep constantly in mind that sleep can be learned.

10. Sleep Analysis Questionnaire

Working out your typical sleep pattern

In the following proposal for making an individual sleep analysis, we have drawn up a list of questions that seem essential for working out a typical sleep record. Anyone, however, can add questions relevant to his own situation. The essential step is to abandon the fatalistic assertion, "I just can't sleep," and to arrive at the active assertion, "I am going to learn it again," and to accomplish this by self-examination and by the conscious use of information relevant to oneself.

The test should be taken over a period of at least one week, preferably two weeks. You can simplify matters for yourself by taking plenty of time. Keep the questionnaire conveniently within reach so you will not forget to write down your observations. The questionnaire is not a test in the sense of answering questions with yes or no to win points, showing that you are a good or a bad sleeper. You know that from the outset. The result should provide you with an insight into pattern of living and show it in relation to your sleep habits. Carefully search for and observe all your attitudes and all the external conditions and activities that improve your sleep. Try to find an increasing number of plus factors that lay the groundwork for you to sleep well.

117

Enter here within the next two weeks what you are able to observe about your sleep or about your partner's sleep. It will enable you to get to know your typical pattern of sleep, which is the first condition for learning to sleep well again.

1. When did I go to bed? Specific time?	
a. Did I still read in bed?	
b. Did I still discuss any important problems with my partner?	
c. Were we in a good mood?	
d. Were we cross about anything?	
e. Did we have sexual contact?	
f. How much time elapsed before the light was turned out?	
2. How long did I (subjectively) lie awake?	
3. Did I check the amount of time by the clock or did I just estimate it?	
4. Did I sleep through the night?	
5. If not, how often did I wake up?	
6. When did I wake up?	

7. Can I recall a dream?

8. What time did I wake up in the morning?

9. How many hours did I sleep?

10. How much time elapsed between waking up and getting up?

11. How did I feel—done in, tired, bad-tempered, depressed, passive, indifferent, happy, refreshed, energetic?

12. Did I sleep alone or with my partner?

13. Did my partner sleep well?

14. Did my partner snore?

15. Did my partner disturb me in any other way?

16. Were there any additional, unfamiliar sources of disturbance during the night?

17. How long did my partner sleep?

18. Was I glad my partner had slept well, or was I envious?

19. How did I spend the morning?

20. Did I feel productive or exhausted in the morning?

21. Was I tired or fresh at noon?

22. Did I work during the noon break, or did I lie down?

23. Did I sleep for a short while during the noon break? Or for a longer period?

24. Was I out in the fresh air during the course of the day?

25. Did I drink coffee or tea?

26. If so, when?

27. Did I drink any alcohol?

28. If so, what and when?

29. Did I take any medications?

30. If so, when and which ones?

31. How did I spend the afternoon?

32. When did I eat dinner?

33. What did I eat for dinner?

34. How did I spend the evening? Did I go out? Read? Watch TV? Was I occupied with professional matters? Personal matters? A hobby? Did I work in the garden? Go to the movies or theater?

35. Did I have any aggravations at work?	
36. Do I have any worries about the family?	
37. Do I have financial worries?	
38. Did I quarrel with anyone?	
39. Was I particularly happy about anything?	
40. Am I preoccupied with a problem that cannot be solved in the immediate future?	

Index

HEALTH & CURE SERIES

Positive Family Therapy: The Family as Therapist
M.D. Nossrat Peseschkian, 1995, ...1839 9, 352pp, Rs. 150

Psychotherapy of Everyday Life: Training in Partnership and Self Help with 250 Case Histories
M.D. Nossrat Peseschkian, 1995, ...1838 0, 264pp, Rs. 125

Oriental Stories as Tools in Psychotherapy
M.D. Nossrat Peseschkian, 1992, ...1071 1, 184pp, Rs. 95

Stress Management: Through Yoga and Meditation
Pandit Shambhunath, 1993, ...1514 4, 198pp, Rs. 70

You and Your Medicines
R.R. Chaudhary, 1994, ...1588 8, 120pp, Rs. 50

Overcoming Anxiety
G.K. Sahasi & H.M. Chawla, 1993, ...1461 3, 56pp, Rs. 25

The Pregnant Year: A Motherhood Diary
Monika Datta, 1994, ...646 9, 204pp, Rs. 99

Stress: An Owner's Manual
Arthur Roshan, 1994, ...1673 6, 160pp, Rs. 70

Yoga, Meditation and The Guru
Purusottama Bilimoria, 1993, ...1478 4, 104pp, Rs. 45

SPEAKING OF

Alternative Medicine Acupuncture
Drs. Nilesh Baxi & C.H. Asrani, 1994, ...1774 0, 112pp, Rs. 50

Ayurvedic Remedies for Common Diseases
Dr. T.L. Devaraj, 1993, ...1611 6, 152pp, Rs. 60

Child Care—Everything you wanted to know
Dr. Suraj Gupte, 1995, ...1795 3, 232pp, Rs. 80

Heart Attacks
Drs. Carola Halhuber, Max. J. Halhuber, 1987, ...0261 1, 128pp, Rs. 60

Yoga and Nature Cure Therapy
K.S. Joshi, 1993, ...1360 5, 158pp, Rs.50

Sleeping Problems
Dr. Dietrich Langen, 1995, ...1773 2, 128pp, Rs. 50

Diabetes and Diet
Deepa Mehta, Dr. S.A. Vali, 1993, ...1048 7, 128pp, Rs. 45

Fitness Over 40
Dr. Walter Noder, 1995, ...1796 1, 128pp, Rs. 55

Asthma
Dietrich M.D. Nolte, 1988, ...0841 5, 96pp, Rs. 35

Healing Through Gems
N.N. Saha, 1992, ...0054 6, 144pp, Rs. 70

Nature Cure
L. Sarma & S. Swaminathan, 1995, ...0632 3, 232pp, Rs. 70

Yoga—A Practical Guide to Better Living
Pandit Shambhunath, 1995, ...1794 5, 198pp, Rs. 70

High Blood Pressure
Dr. Hanns P. Wolff, 1995, ...1772 4, 128pp, Rs. 50